100 Questions & Answers About Hepatitis C:
A Lahey Clinic Guide

Stephen C. Fabry, MD
Senior Staff Physician
Gastroenterology and Hepatology
Lahey Clinic Medical Center
Assistant Professor of Medicine
Tufts University School of Medicine

R. Anand Narasimhan, MD
Senior Fellow in Gastroenterology
Lahey Clinic Medical Center
Clinical Instructor of Medicine
Tufts University School of Medicine

JONES AND BARTLETT PUBLISHERS
Sudbury, Massachusetts
BOSTON   TORONTO   LONDON   SINGAPORE

World Headquarters

Jones and Bartlett Publishers
40 Tall Pine Drive
Sudbury, MA 01776
978-443-5000
info@jbpub.com
www.jbpub.com

Jones and Bartlett Publishers
Canada
6339 Ormindale Way
Mississauga, Ontario L5V 1J2
CANADA

Jones and Bartlett Publishers
International
Barb House, Barb Mews
London W6 7PA
UK

Jones and Bartlett's books and products are available through most bookstores and online booksellers. To contact Jones and Bartlett Publishers directly, call 800-832-0034, fax 978-443-8000, or visit our website www.jbpub.com.

Substantial discounts on bulk quantities of Jones and Bartlett's publications are available to corporations, professional associations, and other qualified organizations. For details and specific discount information, contact the special sales department at Jones and Bartlett via the above contact information or send an email to specialsales@jbpub.com.

The authors, editor, and publisher have made every effort to provide accurate information. However, they are not responsible for errors, omissions, or for any outcomes related to the use of the contents of this book and take no responsibility for the use of the products and procedures described. Treatments and side effects described in this book may not be applicable to all people; likewise, some people may require a dose or experience a side effect that is not described herein. Drugs and medical devices are discussed that may have limited availability controlled by the Food and Drug Administration (FDA) for use only in a research study or clinical trial. Research, clinical practice, and government regulations often change the accepted standard in this field. When consideration is being given to use of any drug in the clinical setting, the health care provider or reader is responsible for determining FDA status of the drug, reading the package insert, and reviewing prescribing information for the most up-to-date recommendations on dose, precautions, and contraindications, and determining the appropriate usage for the product. This is especially important in the case of drugs that are new or seldom used.

Production Credits
Executive Publisher: Christopher Davis
V.P., Manufacturing and Inventory Control: Therese Connell
Production Director: Amy Rose
Associate Editor: Kathy Richardson
Production Assistant: Jamie Chase
Associate Marketing Manager: Laura Kavigian
Composition: Northeast Compositors, Inc.
Cover Design: Kate Ternullo
Cover Image: © Lee Morris/ShutterStock, Inc.
Cover Image: © Photodisc
Printing and Binding: Malloy
Cover Printing: Malloy

Library of Congress Cataloging-in-Publication Data
Fabry, Stephen.
  100 questions and answers about hepatitis C : a Lahey Clinic guide / Stephen Fabry and R. Anand Narasimhan ; series editor, Andrew S. Warner.
     p. cm.
  Includes bibliographical references and index.
  ISBN-13: 978-0-7637-4077-1
  ISBN-10: 0-7637-4077-2
  1. Hepatitis C—Miscellanea. 2. Hepatitis C—Popular works. I. Narasimhan, R. Anand. II. Title. III. Title: One hundred questions and answers about hepatitis C.
  RC848.H425F33 2006
  616.3'623—dc22

                                    2006014575

6048

Printed in the United States of America
10 09 08 07 06   10 9 8 7 6 5 4 3 2 1

This book is dedicated to our families.

Contents

Contents

Hepatitis C is a significant and growing problem in the United States and throughout the world. At least 4 million people in the United States have been exposed to this virus, and the majority of these people have a chronic infection. A small but significant percentage of patients with chronic hepatitis C will develop cirrhosis; unfortunately, many of these individuals will eventually die of liver failure and liver cancer. Today, hepatitis C is the most common indication for liver transplantation in many transplant centers. Doctors have become increasingly conscientious about screening for hepatitis C in patients with known risk factors for this disease. This effort has led to a huge increase in the number of diagnosed cases, although many patients with hepatitis C remain unaware of their condition. Treatment options have improved significantly over the last decade, with the overall cure rate now exceeding 50 percent. Nevertheless, the management of patients with hepatitis C is complex and requires many complicated decisions to be made. Doctors realize that each and every patient has a unique medical and personal situation that requires careful decision-making. The care of patients with hepatitis C is clearly better when patients take an active role in this decision-making process.

We wrote this book for patients who are interested in becoming involved in this process. We are busy clinicians so we based this book, not only on the medical literature, but also on our personal experiences with patients. Over the years, we have been impressed with the amount of research that some patients pursue on their own. When we were first asked to write this book, we reviewed many other published books and found that those books did not provide the directed and in-depth medical information that is available in our book. Many of these other books were very general and discussed several different types of liver disease. Some focused primarily on the emotional aspects of hepatitis C, with few pages being devoted to discussing the medical facts. We have attempted to write a book that will allow patients to quickly find and understand the answer to any question they have about hepatitis C. We have filled the book with hard medical facts and references to major studies, but have filtered the information to make it more understandable. We have also addressed some of the emotional aspects of this disease and highlighted some alternative therapies. We are confident that this book will help patients better understand hepatitis C and make more informed medical decisions.

Stephen C. Fabry, MD
R. Anand Narasimhan, MD

Hepatitis C is a devastating condition both physically and psychologically. It typically infects individuals without producing any symptoms and then silently damages the liver over many years, sometimes being discovered only after it has resulted in cirrhosis. Depending on the genotype, hepatitis C can be poorly responsive to therapy, and all of the currently available therapies have significant side effects and toxicity.

It is important for patients who are diagnosed with hepatitis C to have access to clear information regarding their condition. It is often difficult for patients to know which questions to ask or where to turn to have those questions answered accurately.

In this new book, Dr. Stephen Fabry and Dr. R. Anand Narasimhan, respected hepatologists with extensive experience in treating hepatitis C, provide patients with a place to turn. They have done a remarkably thorough job of anticipating questions that patients diagnosed with hepatitis C should want to have answered and have answered each of those questions in a clear and concise fashion. This book is essential reading for patients with hepatitis C who are seeking help in understanding their condition.

Daniel S. Pratt, MD
Executive Director, Liver-Biliary-Pancreas Center
Massachusetts General Hospital
Harvard Medical School

PART ONE

The Basics

Can you give me an overview of the liver and liver disease?

What is hepatitis C?

Who should be screened for hepatitis C?

More . . .

1. Can you give me an overview of the liver and liver disease?

The liver is an amazing and vital organ. The largest organ in the body, it is located on the right side of the abdomen underneath the rib cage (Figure 1). The average person's liver weighs between three and five pounds. Everyone is born with only one liver, so it is important to keep it functioning well. The liver performs many essential functions that are necessary for life. These functions include removing poisons and

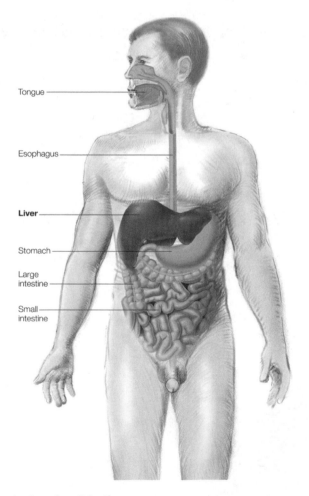

Tongue

Esophagus

Liver

Stomach

Large intestine

Small intestine

Figure 1   Location of the Liver

drugs from the body, manufacturing many different types of proteins, storing energy, fighting infections, storing iron reserves, storing minerals and vitamins, and producing **bile** to help digest food.

The liver processes almost all foods, drugs, and toxins that enter the body into either safer or more usable substances. It produces many proteins, including clotting factors, **albumin** (which accounts for most of the protein in blood), and a variety of proteins that are used as transporters and receptors throughout the body. The liver serves as a major site of energy storage that can be tapped by other parts of the body when necessary.

Liver disease is very common in the United States. Approximately 25,000,000 Americans have a liver-related disorder, including 3.9 million people with **hepatitis** C. About 27,000 Americans die each year from **chronic** liver diseases, including as many as 10,000 people with hepatitis C. An estimated 26,000 new infections with hepatitis C and an estimated 60,000 new infections with hepatitis B occur each year.

To keep your liver healthy, you can take several simple steps. Be aware that alcohol can injure the liver either on its own or in combination with a liver disease such as hepatitis C. Because many medicines can affect the liver, it is important to monitor the liver when you are taking certain medications. This monitoring usually consists of blood tests, but occasionally a **liver biopsy** is necessary. You should also inform your doctor of any preexisting liver problems before you begin taking a new medicine. Chemicals, fatty foods, and obesity can also harm the liver.

Bile
greenish fluid produced by the liver that contains bilirubin, bile salts, cholesterol, and lipids. Bile flows through the bile ducts into the intestines, where it helps digest food.

Albumin
a protein produced by the liver that accounts for most of the protein in blood.

Hepatitis
inflammation of the liver that causes cell damage.

Chronic
usually refers to a disease that develops slowly and lasts for a long period of time.

Liver biopsy
a test in which a small needle is passed into the liver and a piece of the liver is removed and then examined under a microscope.

The Basics

Risks for contracting hepatitis A, hepatitis B, and hepatitis C are discussed later in this book. Many people should be vaccinated against hepatitis A and hepatitis B, but no **vaccine** against hepatitis C is available right now.

Unfortunately, many liver diseases, including hepatitis C, often have no symptoms and can be difficult to diagnose. There are, however, certain signs and symptoms that you can watch for—yellow eyes or skin, persistently dark urine, light-colored stools, swelling in the abdomen or legs, confusion, bleeding, itching, and fatigue. These problems are usually a marker of more serious liver dysfunction and possibly liver failure.

2. What is hepatitis C?

Hepatitis C is a virus that can cause inflammation and scarring in the liver and lead to liver failure and liver cancer. These complications do not develop in everyone who has hepatitis C. This virus can also affect other parts of the body such as the kidneys and nerves, although complications outside of the liver are very uncommon. Hepatitis C is a relatively new infection in humans. In fact, the growth of the U.S. hepatitis C virus (HCV)–infected population is believed to have begun around 1960. The pattern of spread has been different in other countries. For example, hepatitis C probably spread several decades earlier in Japan than it did in the United States.

The most common routes of transmission are blood transfusions and intravenous drug use. Today, significantly fewer new cases of hepatitis C occur from blood transfusions because blood products are effec-

Vaccine

a preparation of a specific weakened or killed virus or bacterium that is injected into the body to stimulate the immune system.

The liver performs many essential functions that are necessary for life. These functions include removing poisons and drugs from the body, manufacturing many different types of proteins, storing energy, fighting infections, storing iron reserves, storing minerals and vitamins, and producing bile to help digest food.

tively screened for this virus. Instead, most new cases are related to intravenous drug use and the sharing of needles.

Hepatitis C is a single-stranded **ribonucleic acid (RNA)** virus that belongs to the family Flaviviridae and the genus hepacivirus. The virus has three basic parts: the RNA genome or code, a nucleocapsid core protein, and an outer surface protein complex (Figure 2). Hepatitis C is very good at evading the immune system because it mutates rapidly and the envelope protein can change and fool the body's defense mechanisms. Many different strains of hepatitis C exist.

Ribonucleic acid (RNA)

a material inside cells that contains the genetic code for each specific individual. In humans, RNA copies carry the information from DNA out of the cell's nucleus. In the HCV, RNA is the primary code needed for its replication.

The Basics

HCV Viral Components

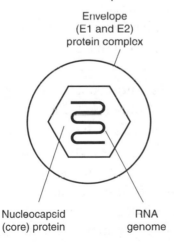

Envelope
(E1 and E2)
protein complex

Nucleocapsid
(core) protein

RNA
genome

Figure 2   The Hepatitis C Virus
Courtesy of the National Digestive Diseases Information Clearinghouse.

Genotype

a major strain of a virus. Because the hepatitis C virus is continually changing or mutating, six major strains of this virus exist.

Hepatitis C is a virus that can cause inflammation and scarring in the liver and lead to liver failure and liver cancer.

The virus can be classified into 6 major **genotypes** and more than 50 subtypes. Genotypes tend to vary geographically; in the United States, the most common genotypes are 1a and 1b. The specific genotype does not significantly alter the severity of disease, but it does affect the likelihood that an infected person will respond to treatment.

3. Who should be screened for hepatitis C?

The medical community has established general guidelines for the screening of diseases. Screening the entire population who might be at risk for a specific disease may be useful for diseases that occur frequently, such as hypertension or colon cancer. Other factors that need to be considered include the ease of the screening test, the cost of the test, the accuracy of the test, and the usefulness of the information gathered. For example, colon cancer screening is recommended for all people over the age of 50 because colon cancer is common, the screening test is relatively safe and accurate, and the identification and removal of polyps decrease the risk of colon cancer.

Screening of the entire population for hepatitis C is currently not recommended, for several reasons. Most patients with hepatitis C have an identifiable risk factor; thus screening of low-risk patients would identify very few people with hepatitis C. Screening tests are not perfect and are more accurate when applied to a population at risk for developing the specific disease. Screening low-risk patients for hepatitis C would result in many "false positive" test results—that is, the test is positive but the patient does not really have hepatitis C. Even though hepatitis C tests are relatively inexpensive, screening the entire population would be prohibitively expensive in terms of the cost per newly identified infection. Current guidelines therefore recommend screening only individuals with an identifiable risk factor.

We can identify people who have a higher risk for acquiring hepatitis C and in whom testing may be more useful. The recommendations for testing include the following groups:

- People with a history of intravenous drug use at any time in their life.
- People who received a blood transfusion, blood products, or an organ transplant before July 1992. (Screening of donated blood for hepatitis C began after this date.)
- Patients with hemophilia who received clotting factors before 1987. (Processing of clotting factors to inactivate viruses began in 1987.)
- Patients with human immunodeficiency virus (HIV) infection.
- Patients with kidney failure on hemodialysis. (Contaminated hemodialysis equipment can place dialysis patients at a high risk for acquiring hepatitis C.)
- Patients with abnormal liver tests.
- Children born to mothers with hepatitis C.
- Anyone who is exposed to hepatitis C–infected blood, such as a healthcare worker after a needlestick injury.
- Sexual partners of patients with hepatitis C.
- Household contacts of patients with hepatitis C.

- All blood donors. (They are screened for hepatitis C to protect the blood supply.)

Anyone with any of these risk factors should ask for a hepatitis C test given the high risk of infection.

4. How many people have hepatitis C?

Antibody

a protein produced by the body's immune system to fight disease.

Cirrhosis

a condition in which normal liver tissue is replaced by permanent scar tissue.

Acute

sudden or severe onset.

Liver transplant

a major surgical procedure that involves the removal of a diseased liver and its replacement with a healthy liver.

Currently, hepatitis C accounts for about 10,000 deaths per year in the United States.

Hepatitis C is a very common infection both in the United States and throughout the world. An estimated 170 million people worldwide are infected with this virus. In the United States, almost 4 million people have a positive **antibody** test. Most of these people have chronic hepatitis C and are at risk for developing **cirrhosis** and subsequent liver failure and liver cancer. Currently, hepatitis C accounts for about 10,000 deaths per year in the United States. This number is expected to increase in the next two decades due to the epidemiology and natural history of this infection. A large number of new infections occurred in the 1960s, 1970s, and 1980s. The peak disease burden from hepatitis C is still ahead of us because progression to cirrhosis can take 20 to 40 years.

Another way to look at the numbers is by noting that hepatitis C accounts for 15 percent of cases of **acute** hepatitis, 60 to 70 percent of cases of chronic hepatitis, and 50 percent of cases of cirrhosis, liver failure, and liver cancer. Roughly half of all **liver transplants** in the United States now involve patients with hepatitis C. This virus is so common that you probably know at least one other person who is infected with it.

5. What can hepatitis C do?

Although hepatitis C can have many effects, it primarily attacks the liver. Most people who are exposed to the virus develop a chronic infection. Many people with chronic hepatitis C develop inflammation in the liver, which can in turn lead to scarring. Severe scarring of the liver, which is called cirrhosis, can lead to liver failure and liver cancer. Fortunately, this progression happens in only about 20 percent of patients with chronic infection. This risk is significantly higher in people who consume excessive amounts of alcohol. Another important point is that patients with cirrhosis do not immediately or even necessarily develop liver failure or liver cancer. Many patients with cirrhosis have an early-stage condition called compensated cirrhosis, in which the liver still functions well and the person can lead a normal life. Patients with HCV-related cirrhosis have a 3 to 4 percent annual risk of developing liver failure and a 1.4 to 6.9 percent annual risk of developing liver cancer. Many of these patients are eligible for liver transplantation. Hepatitis C occasionally leads to problems outside of the liver, including **cryoglobulinemia, glomerulonephritis**, and **porphyria cutanea tarda** (Table 1).

6. Why is hepatitis C so difficult to treat?

Hepatitis C is a particularly difficult infection to treat, although treatments are available and have improved significantly in the last 15 years since the virus was discovered. Treatment limitations are related to both the characteristics of HCV and the medications that are

Cryoglobulinemia

the most common extrahepatic complication of hepatitis C, in which antibodies attack parts of the body and result in skin rashes, joint and muscle pains, and nerve and kidney damage.

Glomerulonephritis

each kidney is made up of tiny structures called glomeruli that produce urine. In this type of kidney disease, the glomeruli are inflamed.

Porphyria cutanea tarda

a blistering skin disease that affects sun-exposed areas of the body due to an enzyme deficiency in the liver. It may be precipitated by hepatitis C infection, iron overload, and alcohol use.

Table 1	Complications of Hepatitis C

Cirrhosis of the liver
Liver cancer
Cryoglobulinemia
Glomerulonephritis
Porphyria cutanea tarda

used to treat the infection. Thanks to research that is providing more information about the virus and new treatment options, we are entering an exciting time in terms of hepatitis C treatment.

Hepatitis C is particularly difficult to treat because the virus changes—that is, mutates—at an incredible rate. As mentioned earlier, there are six major HCV geno-types and many different subtypes. Its constant muta-tions allow the virus to evade the human immune system and establish itself as a chronic infection. These changes also allow the virus to resist therapy in many patients who receive the currently available treatments.

Current treatment options are nonspecific and affect the immune system in a generalized fashion that pro-duces many side effects. As a consequence, hepatitis C is hard to treat because many patients cannot safely take medications or have to stop treatment once side effects develop. Newer treatment options that directly target HCV and cause fewer side effects are under development and should become available within the next 5 years.

7. What should I do now that my doctor says I have hepatitis C?

There are a few things to do when given the diagnosis of hepatitis C. First—and most obviously—do not panic. Panic clouds judgment and can lead to poor decision making. A diagnosis of hepatitis C is not a death sentence. Many patients will never develop severe liver disease, treatments are available, and liver transplantation is an option in severe cases. However, you have just been given a serious medical diagnosis and you have a lot of things to do. Educating yourself is an important step, and reading this book should provide all of the information you need to have productive visits with your doctors. If you are looking for more information, the Internet is another source of almost limitless information. Of course, it is important to approach Internet sites carefully, because many sites have multiple agendas. Government-sponsored sites tend to be unbiased, and many medical groups and organizations also have excellent sites. The "Resources" section at the back of this book lists a variety of useful websites.

Several lifestyle modifications can help patients with hepatitis C. The first and most important step to take is to avoid alcohol. You should also monitor all medications used (including over-the counter [OTC] medicines), maintain a healthy weight, exercise, and eat a healthy diet.

Your doctor will next refer you to a specialist who has more training and experience in dealing with HCV-infected patients. This specialist will be a very important person in your life, so he or she should be someone whom you trust and feel comfortable with.

8. Can you tell me more about lifestyle modifications?

Lifestyle modifications are important for a person's general health in addition to helping with any chronic illness including hepatitis C. A specific question addresses the role of alcohol abstinence more directly, so here we will only say that avoiding alcohol is clearly the most important lifestyle modification that a HCV-infected person can make. You should also completely avoid recreational drugs. This question focuses on diet, exercise, weight control, medications, transmission, and support groups. Some of these issues are also addressed in other parts of the book.

Diet and exercise are increasingly recognized as important components of the management of many diseases and should be part of the overall approach a person takes to deal with hepatitis C. The benefits of diet and exercise are indirect, however, in terms of their effects on HCV. A healthy lifestyle will make you feel stronger, decrease your fatigue and depression, and help you tolerate the side effects of treatment better.

You should eat a normal, healthy, balanced diet. Recent guidelines recommend increasing your consumption of fresh fruits and vegetables, whole grains, and leaner meats and fish and minimizing your intake of processed foods, fats, and low-value carbohydrates.

Regular exercise can improve your physical and emotional condition by reducing stress, decreasing fatigue, and improving the function of the heart and lungs. It may even improve the function of your immune system.

Diet and exercise will also help control any weight problems that you may have. Obesity is increasingly recognized as an independent risk factor for liver disease and as an issue in patients with hepatitis C. **Non-alcoholic fatty liver disease** is the medical term for liver disease secondary to excessive fatty deposition; this condition is often a result of obesity. Hepatitis C treatments are less effective in patients who are overweight. Clearly, controlling your weight is important for many different reasons.

The liver is involved in the processing of almost all medications. Anyone with hepatitis C should be careful with new prescription medications and even OTC medications. Patients without cirrhosis can safely take most— but not all—prescription and OTC medications. Patients with cirrhosis need to be especially careful with their medications. Some common OTC medications, such as acetaminophen (found in Tylenol) and ibuprofen (found in Motrin and Advil), can be very harmful in patients with cirrhosis.

Hepatitis C can be spread sexually, although the risk is very low. Current guidelines call for patients with multiple sexual partners to practice "safe sex" with a condom to reduce the risk of transmission of hepatitis C and other sexually transmitted infections such as HIV and hepatitis B. Patients in a monogamous relationship do not necessarily need to change their sexual practices. Spread of hepatitis C to a partner

The Basics

Non-alcoholic fatty liver disease

liver disease secondary to excessive fatty deposition, often as a result of obesity.

in a stable, monogamous relationship occurs very rarely. We always recommend screening of the partner when we first evaluate a new patient with hepatitis C and the partner is almost always negative unless he or she has other risk factors for acquiring hepatitis C.

Finally, support groups are available throughout the United States. Many people find them helpful for dealing with the emotional issues of a new diagnosis of hepatitis C or the many stresses of living with hepatitis C. Support groups can help you see that you are not alone and allow you to meet other people who are coping with hepatitis C. These groups can give you an outlet for your feelings and frustrations. They also allow hepatitis C patients to share information, compare notes, and help one another.

PART TWO

Transmission

What are the most common risk factors for hepatitis C?

How can I prevent transmission of hepatitis C to other people?

Can hepatitis C be spread through sexual contact?

More...

9. What are the most common risk factors for hepatitis C?

Although there are many potential risk factors for the transmission of hepatitis C, breaching the skin and infecting the bloodstream is the most common way that a person contracts the virus. Consequently, intravenous drug use (IVDU) and blood transfusions are the two most common routes of infection. A history of IVDU is the most likely cause of infection in 60 percent of newly identified cases. In people with a history of IVDU, the risk of hepatitis C increases with the number of injections and the sharing of needles. Hepatitis C infection is also associated with the use of intranasal cocaine, with the virus being spread from blood on shared straws.

Blood transfusions were a common route of transmission until the virus was identified in the late 1980s and blood screening tests were developed for it. The risk of contracting hepatitis C from a transfusion dropped significantly after the routine testing of donated blood began. The current risk is approximately 1 in 100,000. Thanks to newer technology, the risk should be reduced to 1 in 1,000,000 in the near future.

Intravenous drug use (IVDU) and blood transfusions are the two most common routes of infection.

Other risk factors for hepatitis C infection include infusion of clotting factor concentrates before 1987, organ transplantation prior to 1992, exposure to contaminated medical equipment such as hemodialysis equipment, occupational exposure to blood such as healthcare workers with needlestick injuries, sexual activity that involves blood-to-blood contact, tattoos done without proper cleaning of equipment, maternal–fetal transmission, and shared personal care items.

10. How can I prevent transmission of hepatitis C to other people?

Anyone with hepatitis C should be careful about spreading the infection to other people. Viruses are spread through a variety of routes, and each virus has different risk factors for its transmission. For example, hepatitis A and E are transmitted through a "fecal-oral" route. In fecal-oral transmission, the infectious organisms enter the body through ingestion of contaminated food and water. The organisms usually multiply in the digestive system, exit the body through feces, and spread where poor sanitation allows contamination of food or water. Hepatitis A outbreaks, for instance, are commonly traced to food preparers with hepatitis A who have not adequately cleaned their hands. Hepatitis C virus (HCV) is spread through blood-to-blood contact in which HCV-infected blood comes in contact with another person's bloodstream. People with hepatitis C therefore need to be careful about exposing others to their blood.

As mentioned earlier, IVDU is the major risk factor for hepatitis C. Obviously, the most effective way to prevent the virus's transmission would be to enroll in a substance abuse program and stop using drugs. If you have made the decision to continue using drugs, never share syringes or needles with anyone else and use only sterile syringes and needles with a new alcohol swab.

Hepatitis C can be spread through sexual activity only if there is blood-to-blood contact. Patients should inform sexual partners of their infection and the risk of transmission. Individuals in monogamous relationships can discuss this issue with their doctors and decide on the appropriate precautions. Patients who are sexually active with multiple partners should always use a new latex condom with lubricants to reduce the risk of bleeding. This practice will protect against the spread of hepatitis C and other infections that can be transmitted sexually. Hepatitis C patients should never donate sperm, ova, or blood.

Patients should always inform their doctors and dentists about their hepatitis C diagnosis. In addition, healthcare workers should routinely wash their hands before and after every patient contact. Needles and other sharp instruments that have been exposed to patient blood are always handled carefully and discarded into special trash receptacles. Although there have been some reported cases involving possible transmission of HCV between patients who have shared instruments or supplies in dental and medical offices, they are very rare.

Blood must be cleaned thoroughly if it spills, because HCV can live for as long as 4 days on different surfaces. Bloodstains should be cleaned with a bleach solution consisting of 1 part bleach and 10 parts water. At home, do not share razor blades, toothbrushes, nail clippers, or other personal hygiene items with any family members; small amounts of blood on these items may spread infection to others. Always dispose of used feminine hygiene products in plastic bags (Table 2).

Hepatitis C is not spread through casual contact so the sharing of cups, plates, and utensils is felt to be safe.

Table 2   Preventing Spread of Hepatitis C

Stop intravenous drug use

Be aware of the risk of spread through sexual contact

Do not donate sperm, ova, or blood

Clean blood spills appropriately

Do not share razor blades, toothbrushes, nail clippers, etc.

Dispose of feminine hygiene products in plastic bags

Hepatitis C is not spread through hugging and kissing.

11. Can hepatitis C be spread through sexual contact?

The risk of sexual transmission of hepatitis C is very low. One study evaluated approximately 900 people who were partners of patients with hepatitis C. During a 10-year follow-up period, three of these people developed hepatitis C. However, all three had different types of hepatitis C than their partners, suggesting that sexual transmission was not the route of infection in their cases.

Despite this study, you should still be cautious and consider using a condom and lubricants as a matter of course. Because hepatitis C is spread most efficiently from blood-to-blood contact, the risk of transmission is higher when blood is present. In particular, the risk of transmission is increased during "rough" sexual activity or unprotected anal intercourse, where small skin injuries may allow blood-to-blood contact. The risk of sexual transmission is probably higher in certain groups, such as prostitutes and people with multiple

Transmission

sexual partners. Hepatitis C does not appear to be spread through oral sex.

Most doctors recommend testing patients' sexual partners at the time of initial diagnosis. This result will give the patient and his or her partner a baseline study. It is very rare for a partner to test positive unless he or she has other risk factors for hepatitis C. Patients with multiple sexual partners should use condoms routinely. The Centers for Disease Control and Prevention does not specifically recommend that a patient with one long-term steady sex partner change his or her sexual practices after receiving a diagnosis of hepatitis C.

12. Can hepatitis C be spread through household contact?

Hepatitis C is rarely spread through household contact. Despite this, you should be cautious about possible exposures that can spread the virus, perhaps screening all household contacts at the time of initial diagnosis. In terms of household risks, remember that hepatitis C is most efficiently transmitted via blood-to-blood contact. Razor blades, toothbrushes, nail files, and other personal items may have small amounts of blood on their surfaces. There is potential risk of transmission of the virus to other members of the household if a patient with hepatitis C has used these items.

Hepatitis C cannot be transmitted through saliva. Touching, hugging, and kissing are safe. The virus also will not be spread through coughing, sneezing, sharing food and drinks, or in bathrooms.

13. Can I still get hepatitis C from a blood transfusion?

A blood transfusion is the transfer of blood products from one person to another. It may be performed during emergency situations such as surgery or uncontrolled bleeding.

It was a long time before hepatitis C was identified as a specific virus and, unfortunately, many people who donated blood were infected with the virus before testing became available. For many years, the risk of contracting hepatitis C at the time of a blood transfusion was as high as 10 to 15 percent. This risk dropped in the 1980s when donated blood began to be routinely tested for human immunodeficiency virus (HIV) and hepatitis B virus (HBV). Thus, those with HCV who also had HIV or HBV would be identified. In addition, donated blood with abnormal liver tests (caused by HCV) were rejected. After isolation of HCV, screening tests were developed to assess donated blood for this virus as well. The risk of transmission via transfusion dropped significantly once donated blood was tested specifically for hepatitis C. Currently, the risk of contracting hepatitis C from a blood transfusion is very low—approximately 1 in 100,000. Newer technology will be able to detect even smaller amounts of virus in the blood and reduce the risk to 1 in 1,000,000 in the near future.

14. Can I give hepatitis C to my baby if I am pregnant?

Pregnant women are not at a higher risk than nonpregnant women for contracting hepatitis C.

Therefore, pregnant patients need not be screened for hepatitis C unless they have any of the risk factors previously described.

Hepatitis C can be spread to the baby during childbirth. This risk is approximately 5 percent, and there is no known way to decrease this risk or prevent HCV transmission. The risk of transmitting hepatitis C through pregnancy increases if the mother has a high hepatitis C viral level or is infected with HIV. We do not know whether a vaginal delivery or cesarean section is safer in terms of minimizing the risk of transmission to the baby. If you have hepatitis C and become pregnant, you should find an obstetrician who has experience with this situation.

Newborns receive antibodies from their mothers to help them fight infections. This transfer of antibodies to the newborn will result in a positive antibody test for hepatitis C immediately after birth. A positive test does not mean that the newborn has been infected with hepatitis C. More sensitive tests that look for the actual virus, such as the HCV ribonucleic acid blood test, must be given to document active infection. (Treatment of hepatitis C in children is addressed in another question.)

15. Can I breastfeed if I have hepatitis C?

Breastfeeding appears to be safe, although this issue is very difficult to study scientifically. The virus can be detected in breast milk, but it is unlikely to cause transmission of hepatitis C to the child. One theory is that the production of acid in the stomach inactivates the virus. However, if the mother has chapped or cracked nipples, blood may be transmitted to the infant. In such cases, breastfeeding should be withheld. It may be reasonable to periodically test an infant while he or she is breastfeeding from an HCV-infected mother.

16. What is the risk of acquiring hepatitis C from a needlestick injury?

Hepatitis C is a significant health risk for any healthcare worker who is exposed to the blood of an infected patient. A person's risk depends on the amount of virus in the blood and the type of tissue that the blood comes into contact with. This risk may be as high as 10 percent with certain exposures. Most exposures to healthcare workers occur with needlestick injuries. Hepatitis C transmission has also occurred when infected blood is splashed into the eyes of a healthcare worker.

After an exposure, two markers of hepatitis C infection are checked: a hepatitis C viral level and a hepatitis C antibody test. The viral level can turn positive within 10 days of exposure and correlates with active infection. Hepatitis C antibodies are usually detected within 1 month of exposure. These tests also provide baseline information about the person who was exposed.

No exact guideline specifies what should happen after an exposure to HCV. Immediate treatment is not always recommended because many people will fight off the infection and not develop chronic hepatitis C after such an exposure. People who acquire the virus but then fight off the infection will have a positive antibody but a negative viral level. A certain percentage of people will develop hepatitis C that becomes chronic, as signaled by a positive antibody and a detectable viral level. The usual approach is to watch these patients for 3 to 6 months to see if they can clear the infection on their own. If the virus is not cleared, treatment should be considered. Treatment of acute hepatitis C is discussed in a separate question.

17. Is there a vaccine to prevent hepatitis C?

A vaccine is a substance meant to help the immune system respond to and resist disease. It usually consists of a small part or a killed version of the organism that is being targeted. The idea is to expose the immune system to the organism in a controlled fashion so that antibodies to the organism form. If the person is later exposed to the real organism, then the immune system will respond immediately and fight off the infection. Viruses are very common targets of vaccines. In fact, vaccines have already been developed for hepatitis A and B.

Unfortunately, there is no vaccine available that targets hepatitis C.

Unfortunately, there is no vaccine available that targets hepatitis C. As discussed earlier, HCV has multiple genotypes and subtypes. The virus also mutates rapidly when replicating itself. These characteristics make it difficult to develop a vaccine that would be effective against HCV. There appears to be little chance of developing a hepatitis C vaccine anytime soon.

PART THREE

Natural History and Symptoms

What is the natural history of hepatitis C?

What are the signs and symptoms of hepatitis C infection?

Can the liver worsen while someone feels well?

More...

18. What is the natural history of hepatitis C?

Hepatitis C usually takes several decades to progress to cirrhosis. This long time course of hepatitis C infection makes it difficult to study groups of patients and develop good models for its natural history. Several groups of people with a known infection source and time (such as tainted clotting factor products) have been followed for decades. In addition, there have been several retrospective (looking backward in time) studies, although this type of medical study tends to be less accurate.

Most people with chronic hepatitis C virus *do not* develop cirrhosis and its complications of liver failure and liver cancer. The following statistics summarize our current best estimates of the natural history of hepatitis C:

- 55–85 percent of persons develop a chronic infection
- 20 percent develop cirrhosis (over a period of 20–40 years)
- 1–5 percent develop liver cancer or liver failure
- approximately 50 percent of liver transplants are done for patients with hepatitis C

Most people with chronic hepatitis C virus do not develop cirrhosis and its complications of liver failure and liver cancer.

Certain factors are associated with a higher risk for developing cirrhosis—most significantly, alcohol use. Other risk factors include an older age at infection, long duration of infection, male sex, human immunodeficiency virus (HIV) coinfection, and other conditions that compromise a person's immune system. The amount of fat in the liver and a person's race may also influence the risk of developing cirrhosis.

19. What are the signs and symptoms of hepatitis C infection?

Most people with hepatitis C infection have no signs or symptoms of liver disease. In medicine, a sign of a disease is a finding noticed by the doctor, while a symptom of a disease is a sensation noticed by the patient. Some patients will experience mild and non-specific symptoms including fatigue, mild discomfort over the liver, nausea, and a poor appetite. It is difficult to confirm that these symptoms are directly related to hepatitis C because they are common in many people without the infection. Similarly, most patients do not have any signs of infection. Once cirrhosis develops, there are subtle signs of early or "compensated" cirrhosis and obvious signs of late or "decompensated" cirrhosis. Signs of early cirrhosis include enlargement of the liver or spleen, spots on the skin, and certain blood test abnormalities. Signs of late cirrhosis include **jaundice**, muscle wasting, abdominal swelling, ankle swelling (**edema**), and confusion (Table 3).

Jaundice

yellowing of the skin and eyes that can occur due to liver disease.

Edema

excess fluid in the body that can cause swelling of the extremities and abdomen

Table 3   Signs and Symptoms of Cirrhosis
Abdominal pain
Exhaustion
Fatigue
Decreased appetite
Nausea
Itching
Easy bleeding & bruising
Jaundice
Palmar erythema
Abdominal swelling
Leg swelling
Confusion

20. Can the liver worsen while someone feels well?

Deterioration of the liver can definitely occur while someone feels well. Although somewhat melodramatic, hepatitis C has been labeled the "silent killer." As mentioned in the previous question, most patients with hepatitis C have no symptoms. Despite feeling well, some of these patients may have active inflammation and progressive scarring in the liver. This damage can continue for decades, so that many people develop cirrhosis without ever experiencing any symptoms. In this situation, the onset of symptoms or signs of hepatitis C usually signifies the development of liver cancer or liver failure. Some patients will develop symptoms earlier in the infection process—either from chronic infection or when cirrhosis first develops.

Hepatitis C needs to be treated before people have signs and symptoms of liver failure because it is dangerous and less effective to treat patients with decompensated cirrhosis.

Many people naturally want to put off treatment until they feel sick. Obviously, waiting until serious problems arise is a very flawed approach to hepatitis C. Hepatitis C needs to be treated *before* people have signs and symptoms of liver failure because it is dangerous and less effective to treat patients with decompensated cirrhosis. Once a person has decompensated cirrhosis, the only long-term option is liver transplantation. The best time to treat a patient is early in the infection, when the person may have no symptoms. Opting for treatment is often a difficult decision to make because the therapy will usually make a person feel much sicker than hepatitis C itself. We would consider this a short-term sacrifice intended to gain a long-term benefit.

21. What is the best way to monitor the liver in hepatitis C?

There are many different ways to monitor the liver in hepatitis C (Table 4). Possible parameters that can be followed include symptoms, liver function tests, viral levels, and liver biopsies. As discussed in the previous question, hepatitis C can worsen while someone feels well, so symptoms are not really a good way to monitor a person's status. Similarly, blood tests, which include liver function tests and viral levels, do not accurately show what is actually going on in the liver. These numbers can remain stable even as the condition of the liver worsens. The results of these blood tests often fluctuate significantly, and the levels do not correlate exactly with what is actually happening in the liver. Patients are often preoccupied with their liver tests and viral levels, so doctors should emphasize that the numbers are an unreliable monitoring tool. Completely normal liver function tests decrease the likelihood that a person will have severe scarring in the liver. However, normal liver function tests do not definitively exclude significant disease.

The best test to monitor the liver is a liver biopsy. (Liver biopsies are discussed in more detail in Part 4,

Table 4 Monitoring Hepatitis C
Liver function tests
Hepatitis C viral level
Liver biopsy

Biopsy

the removal of a small piece of tissue using a thin needle.

"Testing and Evaluation.") A **biopsy** is often done as part of the initial evaluation to help decide on the need for treatment and to serve as a baseline against which to measure any future liver biopsies. While not perfect, a biopsy is considered the gold standard for assessing the amount of inflammation and scarring in the liver. Biopsies are the best way to monitor and follow the liver in patients who are not treated. The usual approach is to repeat a biopsy every 3 to 5 years. The need for treatment can be reassessed if the liver biopsy shows increasing amounts of scarring.

Robert's comments:

After testing positive for HCV, my doctor and I discussed the various options regarding further testing and treatment. We discussed the subject of biopsy at length. I was told that some people opt not to have it done, citing the risks such as internal bleeding. In view of this, I considered the fact that the biopsy would be my only accurate method of knowing the current condition of my liver. If I had not done it, I would have gone through treatment without knowing if there was any permanent damage and it would always have been on my mind.

22. What is the relationship between hepatitis C and alcohol?

In the United States, alcohol consumption is a major cause of chronic liver disease, cirrhosis, and liver failure. Numerous studies have shown that the combination of hepatitis C and alcohol increases the risk of developing cirrhosis. These studies have repeatedly arrived at the same conclusion: heavy alcohol use significantly increases the amount of liver damage in patients with hepatitis C, and light alcohol use leads to milder increases in liver damage. The implication of these studies is both simple and obvious: patients with hepatitis C should not drink alcohol.

Active alcohol use is also considered a relative contraindication to treatment. Most doctors require abstinence before they will undertake a liver biopsy and begin treatment for several reasons. Active alcohol use leads to liver inflammation and can confound liver biopsy interpretation. Liver biopsy interpretation will be more meaningful in a patient who has refrained from using alcohol for an extended period of time. Current **interferon**-based regimens have multiple side effects and require close follow-up. Most doctors feel that a patient with active alcohol use will have a more difficult time assessing side effects and committing to the follow-up required during treatment. Ideally, patients should be abstinent and involved in an alcohol treatment program before they start hepatitis C therapy.

Active alcohol use is also a contraindication to liver transplantation. Transplant programs require at least six months of complete abstinence, and many programs also require active involvement in an alcohol treatment program.

Robert's comments:

The results of my biopsy indicated I had liver fibrosis at a stage of 2–3 (on a scale of 4). Although there is no way to be certain, I feel sure the combination of moderate to heavy alcohol use along with the virus was primarily responsible

Interferon

a family of proteins that are naturally produced by the body and that fight off infection. There are three types: alfa, beta, and gamma. Alfa-interferon is used to treat hepatitis C.

Numerous studies have shown that the combination of hepatitis C and alcohol increases the risk of developing cirrhosis.

for this staging, and that my liver condition would have been much better had it just been the virus alone.

23. Are there patient risk factors other than alcohol that cause hepatitis C to progress quickly?

Hepatitis C has a variable natural history, but certain factors appear to influence a person's risk of developing fibrosis and cirrhosis (Table 5). Established risk factors other than alcohol intake include male sex, older age of infection (older than 40 years), longer duration of infection, hepatitis B virus (HBV) coinfection, and HIV coinfection. Other immunocompromised conditions, including organ transplants, are also associated with increased rates of fibrosis. This risk is a major issue in patients who receive a liver transplant for hepatitis C. Other risk factors for the development of cirrhosis that are being investigated include the amount of fibrosis on liver biopsy, the amount of fatty tissue on liver biopsy, and race.

Table 5   Risk Factors for Developing Cirrhosis
Alcohol consumption
Infection at older age
Long duration of infection
Male sex
HIV coinfection
Hepatitis B coinfection
Immunocompromised conditions
Fatty liver

Your doctor will assess all of these risk factors when making a decision about your treatment. Some risk factors are obvious—for example, your age and sex. In addition, your history may give clues about when you acquired hepatitis C and how long you have had the infection. Tests for HBV and HIV can be performed at the initial evaluation. A liver biopsy will grade the amount of inflammation and scarring in the liver. Modifiable risk factors, including alcohol use and obesity, need to be treated aggressively. These factors, used in conjunction with other information, will help your doctor decide on the correct treatment for you.

24. Can hepatitis C lead to problems outside the liver?

Although hepatitis C can lead to complications outside the liver, such problems happen in only 1 to 2 percent of HCV-infected people. The most common **extrahepatic** (not in the liver) complication is cryoglobulinemia, in which a person develops antibodies that attack other parts of the body. A patient with cryoglobulinemia can develop skin rashes, joint and muscle pains, nerve damage, and kidney damage. Other extrahepatic complications include another type of kidney disease called glomerulonephritis and a skin disease called porphyria cutanea tarda. Although some other diseases may have an association with hepatitis C, the scientific data proving these links remain sketchy.

Extrahepatic
A term used to refer to organs other than the liver.

It is important to be aware of these extrahepatic complications because treatment for hepatitis C may help prevent these diseases. Patients are sometimes sent for

HCV treatment when hepatitis C is diagnosed and felt to be the cause of the patient's kidney disease. In these patients, treatment is often indicated only for the extrahepatic complication and not to prevent liver damage.

PART FOUR

Testing and Evaluation

Can you give me an overview of testing
and evaluation?

What is a hepatitis C antibody test?

What is a direct test for the hepatitis C virus?

More...

25. Can you give me an overview of testing and evaluation?

Your doctor can test and evaluate you for hepatitis C, the function of the liver, and the presence of other liver diseases in several different ways. The standard test for hepatitis C is an antibody test, which looks for evidence of antibodies to hepatitis C. In a patient with a risk factor for hepatitis C and abnormal liver function tests, a positive antibody test is almost always a sign of chronic hepatitis C. In confusing cases or when the doctor wants to confirm a diagnosis, the hepatitis C viral level can be checked. This test looks for the actual virus and can estimate how many viral particles are present. A viral level and a genotype test are also checked before treatment.

Liver function tests consist of a general panel of tests that are checked for many different reasons. They are typically performed while screening a patient with a risk factor for hepatitis C or for another medical problem. If the liver function tests are abnormal, then additional tests for hepatitis C and other liver diseases are performed. If a diagnosis of hepatitis C is already established, then liver function tests can provide a general sense of how much inflammation and scarring are present in the liver.

Liver function tests are not perfect—they do not always reflect what is actually happening in the liver. Other tests that help assess the amount of inflammation and scarring in the liver include imaging studies such as an **ultrasound** and liver biopsy. An ultrasound can provide clues that suggest more advanced scarring

Ultrasound

a diagnostic test that uses sound waves to evaluate internal organs.

and can look for tumors, which sometimes develop in patients with hepatitis C. A liver biopsy is the best test for assessing the amount of inflammation and scarring in the liver.

Your doctor will also test you for other types of liver diseases. Hepatitis A and B tests are routinely checked. Patients who are diagnosed with hepatitis C should be vaccinated against hepatitis A and B if they are not already immune to these viruses. **Autoimmune hepatitis** and **hemochromatosis** should be excluded in patients with hepatitis C because the presence of either disease would significantly alter the management of hepatitis C.

26. What is a hepatitis C antibody test?

An antibody is a protein produced by the immune system that can identify and attack foreign objects in the body, such as bacteria and viruses. Antibody tests are commonly used to check for either active infection or previous exposure to a specific bacteria or virus. When a person is infected with hepatitis C, the immune system counters the invading virus by producing antibodies against hepatitis C in an attempt to fight off the infection. A positive hepatitis C antibody test usually represents active infection because few people successfully fight off the infection.

The standard hepatitis C virus (HCV) antibody test is an enzyme immunoassay (EIA) test. This test is very accurate when used to screen high-risk populations such as people with abnormal liver function tests or people with clinical signs of liver disease. The hepatitis C EIA test is not perfect, however. False positive

Autoimmune hepatitis

a liver disease characterized by an overactive immune system that attacks the liver.

Hemochromatosis

an inherited disorder characterized by the abnormal accumulation of iron in the liver and other organs.

results are possible, especially when the person being tested has no risk factors for hepatitis C. A recombinant immunoblot assay (RIBA) is a more specific antibody test that is often used to confirm a positive EIA and decrease the risk of false-positive results. A direct test for HCV is used to definitively confirm the presence of active infection (see the next question).

Conversely, antibody tests can be unreliable and produce negative results in patients with active hepatitis C infection. During an acute infection, it takes approximately 4 weeks for the antibody test to become positive. During this period, a direct HCV test should be performed if acute hepatitis C is suspected. Hepatitis C antibody tests may also be falsely negative if the person does not produce enough antibodies for detection with the EIA or RIBA test. This happens in patients with conditions such as human immunodeficiency virus infection or congenital immunodeficiencies where the immune system does not function properly. A direct viral test is necessary in these situations.

27. What is a direct test for the hepatitis C virus?

Direct tests for HCV look for the actual viral ribonucleic acid (RNA) in a patient's blood. These tests can detect even a small amount of virus because the viral RNA is amplified many times. The virus can be amplified by several different methods, including polymerase chain reaction (PCR) and branched deoxyribonucleic acid signal amplification. We will refer to the various direct tests simply as hepatitis C RNA tests or a hepatitis C viral level.

A hepatitis C RNA test can be classified as either a qualitative test or a quantitative test, depending on how the result is reported. A qualitative test is reported as either positive or negative. Because it can detect a very low level of virus, a qualitative test is administered after antiviral treatment is completed to check for a cure. A quantitative test detects not only the presence of virus but also the amount of virus in the blood. Quantitative tests are very helpful during treatment when the viral level is followed closely and used to make decisions about whether treatment should continue.

The PCR assay is the most common RNA test currently used in cases of hepatitis C. The result is reported as either copies per milliliter or international units per milliliter (IU/mL); one international unit is roughly equivalent to two copies. An RNA test is almost always done after a positive antibody test to confirm a new diagnosis of hepatitis C. An RNA test should also be performed in situations where antibody tests are unreliable, such as in cases of acute hepatitis C and in patients with compromised immune systems. The results of a quantitative RNA test are checked immediately before treatment begins. Because the viral level does not correlate with the severity of infection, this level should not be followed as a marker for disease progression. However, the viral level does correlate with the chance of a response to treatment. Patients with a high viral load (usually defined as more than 2 million copies per milliliter) have a poorer response to treatment than do patients with a low viral load. The viral level is followed closely while patients are on treatment.

28. What is a genotype test?

The hepatitis C virus evades the immune system by mutating rapidly. The virus has evolved multiple strains, which are termed genotypes. A patient's genotype can be determined through a blood test. Although the genotype does not influence the severity of disease and the risk of developing cirrhosis, certain genotypes respond to treatment much better than other genotypes. In fact, genotype is a major predictor of response to current treatments for hepatitis C. As a consequence, the genotype test is very important when deciding on whether to treat a patient and how long to continue the therapy.

There are 6 major HCV genotypes and more than 50 subtypes. Different parts of the world have varying predominant genotypes. In the United States, genotype 1 is most common, accounting for about 75 percent of cases. Most of the remaining cases in the United States are genotypes 2 and 3, with an occasional genotype 4 patient. Genotype 4 is the most common genotype in Africa including Egypt, where 18 percent of the population has been exposed to hepatitis C. Genotype 5 is the most common genotype in South Africa, and genotype 6 is the most common in Southeast Asia. Genotypes 7, 8, and 9 are closely related to genotype 6.

Most of the large treatment studies have been done in countries where almost all patients are genotypes 1, 2, and 3, so there are few data on treating patients with genotypes 4, 5, and 6. Genotype 1 is the most difficult to treat, whereas genotypes 2 and 3 tend to respond to treatment significantly better. It is important to know a patient's genotype when making a decision to treat because of these large differences in treatment responses.

29. What are liver function tests?

Liver function tests are laboratory values used to evaluate the functioning of the liver. A variety of blood tests are available to assess the liver, including tests that reflect inflammation in the liver and tests that gauge the functioning of the liver (Table 6). Doctors usually order a standard group of tests called a **liver panel** that includes aspartate aminotransferase (AST), alanine aminotransferase (ALT), **bilirubin, alkaline phosphatase**, and albumin. The **aminotransferase** (AST and ALT) levels reflect the amount of inflammation in the liver, and the albumin and bilirubin levels reflect the functioning of the liver. Alkaline phosphatase levels can rise in many liver conditions, but elevations are especially likely when the bile ducts are blocked.

Liver function tests are not perfect. For example, a person can have a normal aminotransferase level and still have inflammation in the liver; similarly, a patient can have normal albumin and bilirubin levels and still have scarring in the liver. Because of this unreliability, many doctors recommend a liver biopsy even in patients with normal liver function tests. The many different patterns observed with liver function test abnormalities reflect different medical conditions and different levels of functioning in the liver.

Elevated liver function levels can occur in other medical conditions because the enzymes measured by these tests are present in other parts of the body besides the liver. For example, alkaline phosphatase is found in

Liver panel

a standard group of laboratory tests used to evaluate the functioning of the liver. These tests usually measure the levels of aspartate aminotransferase (AST), alanine aminotransferase (ALT), alkaline phosphatase, albumin, and bilirubin.

Bilirubin

a product of the breakdown of hemoglobin that is measured to screen for or to monitor liver or **gallbladder** dysfunction.

Alkaline phosphatase

a blood test that measures injury to the liver or the bile ducts.

Aminotransferases

blood tests that measure enzymes found in liver cells. These levels are often elevated in patients with liver disease. Aspartate aminotransferase (AST) and alanine aminotransferase (ALT) are the two most commonly measured.

Gallbladder

a pouch connected to the biliary system that stores bile.

Testing and Evaluation

Table 6   Liver Function Tests

Liver Function Tests	Normal Values
Total Protein	6–8.2 g/dL
Albumin	3.2–4.8 g/dL
Globulin	2–4 g/dL
AST	11–40 IU/L
ALT	7–40 IU/L
Alkaline Phosphatase	30–115 IU/L
Total Bilirubin	0.2–1.3 mg/dL
Direct Bilirubin	< 0.3 mg/dL

bone and the placenta and can become elevated in bone disease and pregnancy. Likewise, AST is present in many parts of the body, including muscle, and its level will rise whenever muscle is destroyed, such as during a heart attack. These other conditions need to be considered when the patient does not have obvious liver disease.

Aminotransferase (AST and ALT) levels are used to measure direct injury to liver cells. These levels are often—but not always—elevated in patients with chronic hepatitis C. Elevated aminotransferases on routine blood test screening are often the results that lead to the initial diagnosis of hepatitis C. Several different patterns of aminotransferase elevations can be meaningful in patients with hepatitis C:

• Normal levels do not exclude more advanced liver disease, but severe scarring or cirrhosis is less commonly seen in this situation.

- Aminotransferase levels can fluctuate in an individual patient without having a direct correlation with what is actually happening in the liver.
- The ALT level is usually higher than the AST level in patients without cirrhosis. A reversal of this pattern—that is, AST level higher than ALT level—can be a marker for the development of cirrhosis.
- Very high levels (greater than 300 IU/L) should prompt evaluation for other conditions such as autoimmune hepatitis or an acute injury to the liver such as an acetaminophen overdose.
- Aminotransferase levels are followed during treatment, and most—but not all—patients who respond will have an improvement in the levels.
- An elevated ALT level is strongly suggestive of liver disease, whereas an isolated AST elevation can be seen in many conditions unrelated to the liver, including a heart attack and muscle disorders.

As mentioned earlier, the albumin and bilirubin levels that are included as part of a standard liver panel can reflect the functioning of the liver. Another blood test, called the prothrombin time (PT), reflects **coagulation**, or the body's ability to clot, and is also a good marker of liver function. This test is not in a standard liver profile, however.

The liver produces albumin, which is the main protein in blood. A shortage of albumin can lead to problems with fluid balance and the development of free fluid in the abdomen, a condition known as **ascites**. The albumin level falls as liver function deteriorates; as a consequence, many doctors follow albumin levels closely in their patients with liver disease. One of the major

Coagulation

the ability of the blood to clot

Ascites

abnormal fluid accumulation in the abdomen that can develop when the liver does not function properly.

grading systems for patients with cirrhosis uses the albumin level, bilirubin level, and PT to judge how well the liver is functioning. Kidney failure and malnutrition are other major reasons that a person might have a low albumin level.

The liver helps break down old red blood cells into bilirubin, which is then excreted into the bile ducts. In liver disease, the bilirubin level may become elevated because the liver is less efficient at clearing and processing old blood cells. As the bilirubin level increases, a person may develop yellow eyes or skin. This condition, which is called jaundice, is a sign of poor liver function. Blockage of the bile duct, blood disorders, and even a benign hereditary condition called Gilbert's syndrome are other reasons that a person might have a high bilirubin level.

Alkaline phosphatase is an enzyme found mostly in the liver and bone. In particular, it is found in the cells that line the bile ducts of the liver. The bile ducts help drain the liver, so any process that blocks bile ducts can lead to an elevation of the alkaline phosphatase level. The most common conditions that lead to such elevations are gallstones in the bile duct, cancers that block the bile duct, strictures of the bile duct, and liver diseases that attack the bile ducts. A mildly elevated alkaline phosphatase level is a nonspecific marker in a patient with hepatitis C. A very high level should prompt a search for one of the more common conditions that can cause an alkaline phosphatase elevation.

Robert's comments:

I remember having routine physicals prior to 1990 and seeing liver function tests (ALT and AST) that were ele-

vated from time to time. I was told at that time not to worry, as the elevations were not considered too important. In hindsight, it was probably an indication that the virus (and alcohol) was taking its toll. Unfortunately, HCV was not as well understood then as it is now, and it was in the early days of developing a test for it.

30. What is a liver ultrasound?

Blood tests provide a great deal of useful information about the liver but have several limitations, as discussed earlier. To gather even more information about their patients' conditions, doctors order a variety of radiological tests that can visualize the liver and other organs in the abdomen, including the gallbladder, kidneys, spleen, pancreas, and blood vessels. The most common imaging test of the liver—in cases of hepatitis C—is the ultrasound. Computed tomography and magnetic resonance imaging scans are typically performed as follow-up measures when the ultrasound shows an abnormality; these tests are discussed in a later question.

An ultrasound can provide a lot of information about the liver and the severity of a patient's liver disease. When a patient develops cirrhosis, the size and texture of the liver and spleen may change. Patients who are experiencing liver failure may have a buildup of fluid in the abdomen (called ascites). As noted earlier, patients with hepatitis C and cirrhosis are at risk for liver cancer, and an ultrasound can sometimes pick up liver cancer. Ultrasounds are not perfect, however, so they are used in conjunction with other information when assessing a patient's condition.

Your doctor may order an ultrasound for you in many different circumstances. For instance, an ultrasound test may be performed if you have an abnormal liver test. If a person with known liver disease presents with abdominal pain, an ultrasound may be performed to look for abnormalities, such as liver masses or blockages, in the blood vessels that supply the liver. An ultrasound is also useful to guide procedures such as a liver biopsy or a **paracentesis** (a procedure that drains abdominal fluid in patients with ascites).

Paracentesis

a procedure in which fluid in the abdomen is drained with a needle.

If you have an ultrasound, this is what you can expect. First, the technician applies a jelly directly to the skin; it will make the images clearer for the doctor reading the test. Next, the technician passes a smooth transducer over the skin. The transducer produces sound waves that go through your skin and bounce against your internal organs. A computer processes this information to produce images that will appear on the screen. An ultrasound is not invasive, painful, or harmful. It can be performed on an outpatient or inpatient basis and takes less than an hour.

31. What is a liver biopsy?

Evaluation with blood tests and radiological tests provides a lot of information, but looking at actual liver tissue is often helpful and necessary to make a medical decision. A liver **biopsy** is performed in these cases. During a biopsy, a tiny cylinder of tissue is removed; a pathologist then views the sample under a microscope (Figure 3). A liver biopsy can provide critical information about the cause and extent of a patient's liver disease. For example, if a patient presents with abnormal liver tests and a diagnosis is not clear after initial testing, a liver biopsy may be performed to find a diagnosis. A biopsy may help identify causes of liver

Biopsy

the removal of a small piece of tisse using a thin needle.

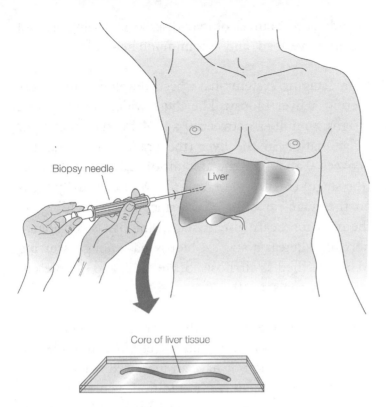

Biopsy needle

Liver

Core of liver tissue

Figure 3   Technique of Liver Biopsy

dysfunction such as drug reaction, autoimmune hepatitis, alcohol use, or cancer for which blood tests and x-rays are often nonspecific.

In hepatitis C, a liver biopsy is usually performed to assess the degree of damage to the liver. If the liver has active inflammation, it can range from mild to severe. Mild disease is characterized by inflammation, but the appearance of liver cells is preserved. As the disease progresses, normal cells are replaced by fibrous tissue. The result may ultimately be cirrhosis, where the liver has scars, nodules (pockets of fibrous tissue), and an irregular appearance. A liver biopsy can also help exclude other sources of liver disease, including alcohol use, iron overload, and autoimmune hepatitis.

Many staging systems have been developed for interpreting a liver biopsy. The most widely used system assigns a number between 0 and 4 for the amount of inflammation in the liver (the grade) and a number between 0 and 4 for the amount of scarring in the liver (the stage) (Figures 4, 5, and 6). Doctors usually focus on the stage (amount of scarring) when deciding on the need for treatment. A stage 0 biopsy is considered normal, whereas a stage 4 biopsy has enough scarring to be classified as cirrhosis. Stages 1, 2, and 3 represent steps between stage 0 and stage 4.

If you have a liver biopsy, this is what you can expect. Your doctor may require you to get blood tests first to ensure that you do not have an increased risk of bleeding after the procedure. In addition, you should discontinue any use of aspirin and aspirin-like products (such as ibuprofen) three to seven days before the biopsy. Ask your doctor about instructions regarding diet. Your doctor may perform the biopsy, or a member of the radiology department may handle the procedure. Initially, your skin will be cleaned with a solution to reduce the risk of infection. Then, the skin is numbed with a medication similar to the novocaine used in a dentist's office. Often, a noninvasive device called an ultrasound is used to guide the procedure. A sample of tissue is removed through a needle and sent to the pathology department for further processing. The biopsy may be performed on an inpatient or outpatient basis. Although it takes less than one-half hour, you will be monitored for several hours afterward.

The most common complication of a liver biopsy is pain. This discomfort usually consists of a dull ache in the right-upper abdomen or shoulder and resolves within 2 hours with or without pain medications. Bleeding, infection, and drug reactions are other less common but potentially serious complications of a biopsy. Unrelenting pain is rare and could indicate a severe complication; notify your doctor immediately if it occurs.

Robert's comments:

The time prior to my biopsy was worse than the actual procedure because of my anxiety. The actual procedure was not that bad. There was some slight pain (more of a slight burning sensation) that extended internally across my abdomen. This pain disappeared after about 2 hours. The recovery time was 3 hours, with about half of that time spent lying on my right side (the entry side of the biopsy). The most important thing for the patient is to discontinue use of blood-thinning products before the biopsy. It is also very important to remain still during the procedure. I believe the biopsy needle passes close to some other organs.

A liver biopsy can provide critical information about the cause and extent of a patient's liver disease.

32. What if I have a positive antibody test but a negative hepatitis C RNA test?

Some patients are screened for hepatitis C and found to have a positive antibody test but a negative hepatitis C RNA test. Several different clinical situations can result in this pattern of testing. First, the antibody test may be wrong. As discussed in a previous question, the standard EIA antibody test sometimes produces false-positive results, especially in patients with no risk factors for hepatitis C. A RIBA antibody test can be performed in this situation. If the RIBA test is negative, the initial EIA antibody test result was most likely a false positive. In this situation, we would recommend rechecking the tests in 3 to 6 months to confirm this finding.

Once a false-positive antibody test has been excluded, several other possibilities need to be considered. A small percentage of patients who are exposed to hepatitis C will successfully fight off the virus. A patient in this situation would have a positive antibody test because of the previous exposure to hepatitis C and a negative RNA test because his or her immune system has successfully cleared the virus. We would consider this possibility strongly in any patient with a known risk factor for hepatitis C. Another possibility in a patient with a known risk factor is that the virus level is so low that the RNA test cannot detect the virus. Studies have shown that viral levels can fluctuate significantly.

It is hard to differentiate between these two situations, although a patient who has successfully fought off hepatitis C would be expected to have normal liver function tests. Patients should be followed closely in both situations, with repeat testing performed on a regular basis. It will become obvious over time which situation applies.

One final scenario to consider is that the patient has been treated successfully for hepatitis C. A careful history will make this fact obvious.

33. What about hepatitis A and hepatitis B?

Hepatitis C is one of many viruses that can cause inflammation of the liver or hepatitis. Other viruses that primarily attack the liver include hepatitis A (HAV), hepatitis B (HBV), hepatitis D, and hepatitis E. Viruses such as cytomegalovirus, infectious mononucleosis, and herpes simplex usually attack other parts of the body but can occasionally cause hepatitis. Hepatitis D is extremely rare and can only infect a person who has chronic hepatitis B. Hepatitis E is similar to hepatitis A but is almost never seen in the United States. Hepatitis A and hepatitis B are the two most important viruses in this group, and every patient with hepatitis C should be tested for these viruses.

HAV is often spread through ingestion of contaminated food or water. Epidemics are common in low-socioeconomic populations where sanitary conditions are less than ideal. Patients may be asymptomatic or may present with jaundice (yellow skin). Almost all patients who are infected with HAV recover fully. An important difference between HAV and HCV is that HAV never causes chronic hepatitis. Treatment of acute HAV consists of rest, fluids, and adequate nutrition; hospitalization is rarely required. HAV can be prevented with proper hand washing, a clean water supply, and adequate sewage disposal.

If a person has been or may be exposed to HAV, an immunoglobulin (antibody preparation) can be administered to him or her to prevent infection. This measure provides temporary protection against hepatitis A. A vaccination against hepatitis A is also available; the vaccine provides longer (possibly lifelong) protection. Patients with hepatitis C are tested for hepatitis A to see whether they are immune to the latter infection. Many patients were exposed to hepatitis A as a child and have a natural immunity to it. If a patient is not immune to hepatitis A, he or she should be vaccinated. This recommendation is based on a study that suggested patients with chronic hepatitis C who are exposed to hepatitis A are more likely to develop liver failure than patients without hepatitis C.

Hepatitis B is spread through blood, sexual contact, use of intravenous drugs, and from mother to child during childbirth. More than half of the world's population has been exposed to or is infected with HBV. Most of these people live in areas where hepatitis B is endemic and are exposed to this virus at birth. Patients who acquire hepatitis B at birth do not develop acute hepatitis; instead, they typically develop a chronic infection. The United States is not an endemic area for hepatitis B, and less than 2 percent of the U.S. population has been infected or exposed to hepatitis B. Most cases in the United States are acquired as an adult.

Patients who are exposed to hepatitis B as adults usually recover completely and do not develop chronic hepatitis. Symptoms of an acute infection may include joint pain, rash, fatigue, decreased appetite, and jaundice (yellow skin). About 5 to 10 percent of people who are exposed as an adult will not clear the virus and will develop chronic hepatitis. Complications from chronic HBV are similar to those seen with hepatitis C—that is, cirrhosis, liver failure, and liver cancer. Treatment of acute HBV is similar to treatment of

HAV and includes rest, fluids, and adequate nutrition. Treatment of chronic HBV is also available; options include interferon and nucleoside/nucleotide analogs that interfere with replication of the virus.

A vaccination for hepatitis B is available and effective in up to 90 percent of people who receive the vaccine. When it was initially developed, the vaccine was given to anyone considered to be at high risk for exposure to hepatitis B or at high risk for a severe infection if exposed. This population included immunocompromised patients, hemodialysis patients, chronic liver disease patients, healthcare workers, injection-drug users, and individuals with high-risk sexual partners. More recently, the vaccine has been used universally, and all children are vaccinated after birth.

Patients with hepatitis C should be screened for hepatitis B for two reasons: for evidence of chronic hepatitis B and for evidence of immunity. Hepatitis B and hepatitis C share some risk factors, so people occasionally are diagnosed with both chronic hepatitis B and chronic hepatitis C. Treatment recommendations are different in this situation. Patients who are not immune to hepatitis B should be vaccinated for the same reason that vaccination against hepatitis A is recommended—that is, a person with chronic hepatitis C who is exposed to hepatitis B has a higher chance of developing liver failure.

34. What about other liver diseases and medications?

Many patients are diagnosed with hepatitis C when they undergo an evaluation for abnormal liver function tests. There is a standard panel of blood tests that are checked in when a patient has abnormal liver function tests. These include tests for viral, metabolic, and immune liver diseases that can lead to abnormal liver function tests. Other patients are screened directly for hepatitis C because they have a risk factor such as intravenous drug use. These individuals are also screened for other liver diseases because some (such as hepatitis B) share the same risk factors and others (such as autoimmune hepatitis or hemochromatosis) change the management of hepatitis C if they are present.

Hemochromatosis is a hereditary disorder characterized by the abnormal accumulation of iron in organs including the liver, pancreas, joints, and heart. It is a relatively common disease in high-risk groups such as patients with a Northern European ancestry. This disorder can lead to cirrhosis, diabetes, abnormal skin pigmentation, arthritis, and heart abnormalities. Patients usually remain asymptomatic before the age of 40 because it takes many years for a person to accumulate enough iron to develop end-organ damage. Individuals with this disease may present with abnormal liver function tests, cirrhosis, liver failure, or liver cancer. Testing for hemochromatosis includes iron studies, genetic studies, and liver biopsy. All patients with hepatitis C should be screened for iron overload because management of the latter condition would involve removal of the excess iron through phlebotomy before hepatitis C therapy begins.

Autoimmune hepatitis is a rare liver disease characterized by an overactive immune system that attacks the liver. It typically occurs in young to middle-aged women who often have other immune disorders such as rheumatoid arthritis and thyroid disease. Diagnosis is difficult; it involves testing for special antibodies and usually requires a liver biopsy. This disease is treated by suppressing the immune system with medications such as steroids and other immunosuppressants. All patients with hepatitis C should be screened for autoimmune hepatitis because interferon can worsen the latter disease by increasing the activity of the immune system. If a person has both hepatitis C and autoimmune hepatitis, the autoimmune hepatitis needs to be treated first and brought under control. If a patient on hepatitis C therapy develops very high aminotransferase levels, the doctor should be suspicious for autoimmune hepatitis and rule out its presence.

Drug toxicity is a common cause of abnormal liver function tests and liver disease. Some medications may cause a reaction that depends on the dose. Others drugs may produce severe toxicity in the liver on a sporadic basis. Antibiotics, cholesterol-lowering medications, pain medications, anesthetics, hypertension medications, and seizure disorder medications have all been implicated as causes of liver disease. The doctor will take a careful medication history to rule out these possibilities.

35. What other tests might be checked in a patient with hepatitis C?

Many other blood tests may be performed in a patient with hepatitis C. The PT, complete blood count, and basic metabolic profile, including kidney function, are routinely checked in all patients. Other, more specialized tests, such as cryoglobulin levels, a gamma GT, and a 5'- nucleotidase, are performed in specific situations.

The PT reflects the blood's ability to clot. This test is a good marker of liver function because the liver manufactures clotting factors. PT values can vary from lab to lab, so this number is always converted to the **international normalized ratio (INR)**, which adjusts for possible lab variation. As the liver fails and produces less clotting factors, the PT and INR values increase. The INR is part of a major scoring system for cirrhosis that is used to place patients on liver transplant lists.

International normalized ratio (INR)

also known as prothrombin time (PT). It reflects the body's ability to clot and is a marker of liver function.

Sometimes, doctors may purposely give medications that elevate the INR. For example, if a patient has an abnormal heart rhythm, artificial heart valve, or history of stroke, he or she may take blood thinners to reduce the risk of stroke. Warfarin (trade name Coumadin) is the blood thinner most often used for this purpose. An increased INR in a patient who is taking warfarin does not necessarily mean that the person has liver disease.

A complete blood count is checked in all patients with hepatitis C. The main tests in this blood panel include the white blood cell count, hematocrit, and platelet count. The platelet count is especially meaningful because it often decreases in patients with cirrhosis. As the liver becomes scarred, blood flow through the liver slows down. This delay leads to congestion and enlargement of the spleen, which can result in a low platelet count. A low platelet count is often the first sign that a patient has cirrhosis or even liver disease. The white blood cell count and hematocrit can also decrease in patients with more advanced liver disease. These levels are especially important to measure when considering treatment because interferon can suppress the bone marrow, which produces all of these blood cells. These levels are followed closely in patients who are receiving treatment for hepatitis C.

A basic metabolic profile is also checked in all patients with hepatitis C. The most important component of this blood panel is the creatinine (a measure of kidney function). The kidney and liver are closely connected, and kidney function is important to assess for several reasons. Hepatitis C can cause kidney problems, which need to be identified immediately. Kidney dysfunction also affects the medications that can be given to treat hepatitis C.

Gamma GT and 5-prime nucleotidase tests are performed when an elevated alkaline phosphatase level is found. An elevation in alkaline phosphatase can be a marker of liver disease but may also signal the presence of bone disease. Gamma GT and 5-prime nucleotidase are liver-specific enzymes whose levels become elevated when the liver is the source of the elevated alkaline phosphatase levels.

Cryoglobulins are antibodies that the body produces in response to hepatitis C but that attack other parts of the body. This test is performed in patients with hepatitis C who have arthritis or kidney disease.

36. What types of doctors are gastroenterologists and hepatologists?

After completing their undergraduate studies and medical school, physicians may receive training in a number of specialties. **Gastroenterologists** and **hepatologists** must first undergo 3 years of internal medicine training. These doctors then complete a

Gastroenterologist

a physician whose area of expertise includes gastrointestinal and liver disorders.

Hepatologist

a physician whose area of expertise includes liver diseases and liver transplantation.

mandatory 3-year fellowship in gastroenterology. During this time, these doctors gain experience in all parts of gastroenterology, including liver diseases.

A hepatologist has completed further training after internal medicine and gastroenterology. This training usually continues for 1 to 2 years after the fellowship ends. Hepatologists concentrate exclusively on patients with liver disease, including liver damage that may be due to viruses, alcohol, autoimmune causes, and drugs. When these patients have severe disease, they may require a liver transplant. Transplant hepatologists are experienced at evaluating these patients for transplant and guiding their therapies after transplant.

After you receive a diagnosis of hepatitis C, you may be referred to a gastroenterologist or hepatologist for further testing, evaluation, and treatment. Both types of physicians can competently take care of you. If a liver transplant is needed, you will meet surgeons who have trained specifically for this problem. Most centers that provide liver transplants have created multidisciplinary teams whose members—nutritionists, social workers, infectious disease specialists, and psychiatrists—complement these physicians.

PART FIVE

Treatment

Can you give me an overview of treatment?

Can hepatitis C be cured, and how is "cure" defined?

What are the potential benefits of undergoing treatment for hepatitis C?

More...

37. Can you give me an overview of treatment?

One of the most important questions for patients with hepatitis C is whether treatment is necessary and appropriate. This decision is never an emergency and should be considered carefully. Because hepatitis C progresses over years and decades, there is never a medical reason to start treatment urgently. There are many different ways to approach this decision. Some patients have already made a definitive decision by the time of their initial consultation with a gastroenterologist or hepatologist. Most patients, however, are confused and spend a long time discussing the risks and benefits of treatment. The decision-making process is different for every patient. The medical facts that are discussed here are applicable to everyone. The way that you assess the facts and the way that treatment fits into the rest of your life (family, work, friends) is always different and makes each decision-making process unique.

Several issues make this a difficult decision to reach. First, most patients with hepatitis C do not progress to cirrhosis and will never develop symptomatic liver disease. Unfortunately, there is no way to predict with absolute certainty who will develop cirrhosis and when that will happen. The best current test is a liver biopsy, but it gives only a snapshot of what the liver currently looks like and is a less than perfect guide. Therefore, many patients who opt for treatment will probably never progress to cirrhosis even without treatment.

Ribavirin

a synthetic antiviral nucleoside used in the treatment of hepatitis C.

Second, current treatment options all have limitations. Therapy with interferon and **ribavirin** is limited by

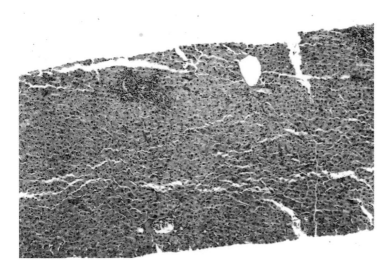

Figure 4   Liver Biopsy: Stage 0

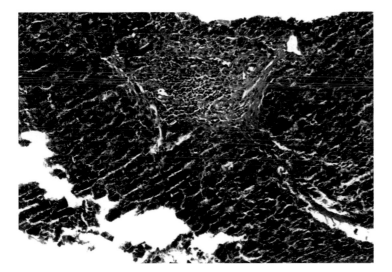

Figure 5   Liver Biopsy: Stage 2

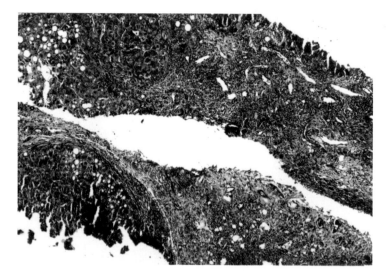

Figure 6   Liver Biopsy: Stage 4

unwanted side effects and variable cure rates, for example. Many patients are not candidates for treatment, and many patients choose to defer treatment because of these concerns.

Patients who do opt for treatment follow a standardized protocol. They take an interferon shot once a week and ribavirin tablets twice a day. The duration of therapy is determined by the viral genotype and the amount of disease found on the initial liver biopsy. The doctor checks the patient's viral levels on a regular basis, and treatment stops if the patient fails to meet predefined goals. Patients are monitored closely for side effects, and treatment is adjusted or stopped as needed. Most studies report overall cure rates of about 50 percent.

Robert's comments:

I feel it is extremely important for patients to do their own research before starting treatment. The Internet has an overwhelming amount of information about this virus, and I feel it is your responsibility to yourself to gather as much information as you find pertinent or that explains topics that are not clear to you. Write it all down, whether or not it may be misleading. You may not understand certain test results, and they will not always be explained if you do not ask. Give your questions and comments to your doctor—it is his or her responsibility to explain them to you. Don't leave without understanding everything because you will need to make decisions based on this information, if you decide to continue with treatment.

Because hepatitis C progresses over years and decades, there is never a medical reason to start treatment urgently.

38. Can hepatitis C be cured, and how is "cure" defined?

A very common question is whether hepatitis C can be cured; the answer depends on the definition of a "cure." The standard definition of a cure in clinical studies is that hepatitis C virus (HCV) cannot be detected in blood tests 6 months after the end of treatment. This outcome is termed a **sustained virological response (SVR)**. Long-term studies have shown that once a person achieves an SVR, the chance of a relapse is very low. The general consensus is that patients who achieve this definition of a cure have a significantly decreased risk of developing cirrhosis or complications of cirrhosis (Figure 7). Treatments have improved sig-

Sustained virological response (SVR)
the standard definition of cure in clinical studies—hepatitis C is not detected in blood 6 months after the end of treatment.

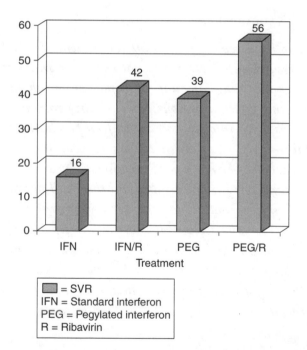

= SVR
IFN = Standard interferon
PEG = Pegylated interferon
R = Ribavirin

Figure 7   Chances of Achieving a Sustained Virological Response with Various Treatments

nificantly over the last decade, and the chance of a cure is significantly higher now than ever before.

39. What are the potential benefits of undergoing treatment for hepatitis C?

This is an important question for anyone considering the currently available treatment regimens with their many potential side effects. We therefore need and have a very good answer for this question: The goal of treatment for hepatitis C is to prevent the development of cirrhosis and the complications of cirrhosis including liver cancer and liver failure. This concept is easy to understand and makes sense. Infection with HCV leads to inflammation in the liver, which leads to scarring, which can eventually lead to cirrhosis. If the virus is removed from the body, the whole process is stopped. Scar tissue is permanent, so the scarring in the liver will remain fixed at the level where it was when the virus was eliminated. Assuming that cirrhosis has not yet developed, the person should have almost no risk of developing liver-related complications in the future.

Unfortunately, large prospective studies that support this argument are not yet available. The problem is that hepatitis C leads to cirrhosis in only a minority of patients, and its progression to cirrhosis usually takes decades. Large groups of patients will need to be studied for long periods of time before we have good scientific support for our theories. Smaller studies and retrospective studies, however, strongly suggest that patients who clear the virus following treatment have lower rates of fibrosis, a lower risk of developing liver cancer, and improved survival.

The standard definition of a cure in clinical studies is that HCV cannot be detected in blood tests 6 months after the end of treatment. This outcome is termed a sustained virological response (SVR).

Treatment

Some studies suggest that even patients with compensated cirrhosis will benefit from treatment. Cure of hepatitis C in a patient with compensated cirrhosis will not eliminate the risk of complications in the future but may significantly reduce the risk, from about 5 percent per year to about 2 percent per year. Successful treatment also has a major benefit in any patient who eventually needs a liver transplant. If the virus is eradicated before the transplant takes place, the risk of hepatitis C recurrence after transplant is much lower.

In general, no treatment is necessary for nonspecific symptoms of hepatitis C such as fatigue and muscle aches. In fact, treatment does not appear to improve these symptoms and is not warranted given its potential side effects. Once safer treatments become available, you might consider trying therapy to see if these nonspecific symptoms improve. An exception is the case in which symptoms are from extrahepatic complications such as cryoglobulinemia or glomerulonephritis. Treatment of hepatitis C can treat these illnesses and is often pursued regardless of the extent of baseline liver injury.

40. What is interferon?

Interferons are a family of proteins that are naturally produced by the body to fight infections. Three classes of interferons exist: alfa, beta, and gamma. Each class has slightly different activities against viruses and bacteria.

Pegylation

the attachment of polyethylene glycol (PEG) to a protein.

Alfa-interferons were first approved by the Food and Drug Administration for treatment of hepatitis C in 1991; they originally required injections three times a week. Modifications since then have produced a longer-acting interferon that can be given just once a week. The initial standard interferons were "**pegylated**" by adding an inactive molecule called polyethylene glycol to them. This alteration changes the way that the body recognizes and destroys the drug and allows the interferon to stay in the body for a longer period of time. As a group, these newer interferons are called **peginterferons**. Two peginterferons are currently available: peginterferon alfa-2b (**Peg-Intron**) and peginterferon alfa-2a (**Pegasys**). The dose of Peg-Intron given depends on the patient's weight and is calculated at 1.5 micrograms per kilogram per week. Pegasys is given as a fixed dose of 180 micrograms per week.

These two interferons appear to have similar effectiveness and side-effect profiles. To date, no large study comparing the two has been published and most gastroenterologists consider them to be equivalent. The major downside to the interferons is that they have many potential side effects.

In addition to the development of peginterferons, the other recent major advance in treatment has been the addition of ribavirin to interferon as part of combination therapy. This leads us to the next question.

41. What is ribavirin?

Ribavirin is a synthetic nucleoside that has antiviral activity. It was first studied in respiratory infections and is approved as a treatment for severe viral pneumonias in infants and young children. Ribavirin was initially studied in hepatitis C as a single-agent therapy but was not effective in eliminating the virus when given by itself. Ribavirin was then combined with standard interferon; this combination resulted in a significant increase in the percentage of patients who had a sustained virological response. Cure rates increased

Peginterferon

a type of interferon in which an inactive molecule called polyethylene glycol is added to standard interferon. This change increases the length of time that the drug remains active against hepatitis C and allows for less frequent injections.

Peg-Intron

a type of peginterferon produced by the pegylation of interferon alfa-2b.

Pegasys

a type of peginterferon produced by the pegylation of interferon alfa-2a.

from approximately 20 percent to 40 percent in three large studies conducted in the 1990s, and ribavirin has been part of standard treatment for hepatitis C since then. When peginterferons were introduced, they were also used in combination with ribavirin.

Ribavirin is generally better tolerated than interferon but does have some potentially significant side effects. Two notable side effects are the development of a severe **anemia** and potential teratogenicity (development of birth defects). Ribavirin can cause serious birth defects, so the patient and his or her partner should not become pregnant while on treatment and for 6 months after the completion of treatment. Patients must use two forms of birth control during this period.

Ribavirin can be dosed either as a fixed dose or as a weight-based dose depending on the viral genotype of the patient being treated.

42. Who should be treated and who should not be treated?

Everyone with hepatitis C should be evaluated for possible treatment. The two major considerations are an individual's risk for developing cirrhosis and liver-related complications and the success rate and safety of the treatment being considered. As yet, there is no model that can predict with complete accuracy a particular patient's risk of developing cirrhosis or decompensation from liver disease. Most doctors depend heavily on the results of the liver biopsy and recommend treatment when the biopsy reveals significant

Anemia
a low red blood cell count.

inflammation and scarring. Some doctors will treat patients with a favorable genotype (2 or 3) without a liver biopsy if the patient is a good candidate and has no contradictions to therapy.

If treatment is felt to be appropriate, patients are carefully assessed to see if therapy can be given safely. Combination therapy with interferon and ribavirin carries many risks, including depression, birth defects, infection, severe anemia, bone marrow depression, thyroid disease, and worsening of an underlying autoimmune disease. Treatment can also worsen quality of life if the patient suffers side effects such as fatigue, flu-like symptoms including fevers and muscle aches, loss of appetite, sleeping problems, and hair loss.

The National Institutes of Health (NIH) held a major meeting several years ago that produced the following guidelines for therapy with interferon and ribavirin:

Absolute Contraindications

Severe or uncontrolled psychiatric disease

Poorly controlled epilepsy

Active serious infection

Pregnancy or inadequate contraception

Severe heart disease

Advanced renal failure

Documented poor compliance

Hemoglobinopathy

Uncontrolled serious medical condition

Relative Contraindications

Hepatic decompensation

Solid-organ transplant (except liver)

Autoimmune disease

Neutrophils $< 0.75 \times 10^9/L$ (low white blood cell count)

Platelet count $< 50 \times 10^9/L$ (low platelet count)

Severe anemia

Ongoing alcohol or substance abuse

Hepatic

a term used to refer to anything pertaining to the liver.

Everyone with hepatitis C should be evaluated for possible treatment.

Your doctor will obviously assess you carefully prior to starting treatment. Further tests—for example, a pregnancy test, stress test of the heart, or psychiatry consult—may be requested by your doctor before therapy begins if he or she has any specific concerns.

43. Can you describe current treatment protocols?

Over the last 15 years, the treatment of hepatitis C has evolved from standard interferon monotherapy (single-agent therapy) to combination therapy with standard interferon and ribavirin to combination therapy with peginterferon and ribavirin. Occasionally, patients with special situations are treated with interferon monotherapy; these patients usually have an absolute contraindication to ribavirin. In this question, we will focus on the standard patient who is treated with combination therapy.

There are two peginterferons on the market: Peg-Intron and Pegasys. Although no study has directly compared the two, studies comparing each to standard interferon and ribavirin resulted in very similar SVR rates for both peginterferons. We will assume for now that they are equivalent and use the generic term peginterferon to apply to whichever one your doctor has chosen. The major decisions, then, are the dose and the duration of treatment. The major factors that influence these decisions are the genotype and the presence (or absence) of cirrhosis.

The peginterferons are given at a standard dose in all patients. Peg-Intron is dosed based on patient weight at 1.5 micrograms per kilogram per week. Pegasys is given as a fixed dose of 180 micrograms per week. Ribavirin is usually dosed based on the genotype. Genotype 1 patients are dosed by weight: 1,000 milligrams daily in two divided doses in patients weighing less than 75 kilograms (165 pounds) and 1,200 milligrams daily in two divided doses in patients weighing more than 75 kilograms. Genotype 2 and 3 patients are usually dosed at a standard 800 milligrams of ribavirin in two divided doses. In some studies, weight-based ribavirin dosing is also used in patients with genotypes 2 and 3. Genotypes 4–7 are rarely seen in the United States. Because data on these genotypes are lacking, patients with these genotypes are usually managed much like genotype 1 patients.

All genotype 1 patients are treated for 48 weeks if they show appropriate viral level responses at weeks 12 and 24. An appropriate drop in viral levels at these time points is termed an **early virological response (EVR)** and is used to decide whether treatment should

Early virological response (EVR)

refers to the appropriate drop in hepatitis C viral levels that determines whether treatment should continue.

continue. The EVR at 12 weeks is a 2-log (100-fold) decrease in the viral level, and the EVR at 24 weeks is an undetectable viral level. In other words, if your viral level has fallen less than 100-fold at the 12-week mark or is still detectable at the 24-week mark, your doctor will probably recommend stopping treatment because the chance of cure or SVR is close to zero. If the viral level is close to the cutoff, some doctors will continue treatment for an extra month to see whether an EVR is reached. If the goal viral level is reached after the extra month, treatment continues and an extra month is added on to the treatment duration at the end. Genotype 2 and 3 patients are usually treated for 24 weeks; their viral levels are not necessarily checked during treatment because of the high cure rates associated with these genotypes.

Doctors may vary how they structure the treatment protocol. Some doctors will continue therapy for harder-to-treat genotype 2 and 3 patients such as cirrhotics for a longer period of time such as 48 weeks. More recently, doctors have been checking viral levels at the 4-week mark. A rapid viral level drop over the first few weeks of treatment appears to correlate with a better overall cure rate. A recent study suggested that patients with genotypes 2 and 3 who have an undetectable viral level at the 4-week mark can be treated for 12 weeks instead of 24 weeks and still have similar SVR rates.

Let's summarize the treatment protocols from the genotype perspective:

• Patients with genotype 1 will be treated with the standard peginterferon dose and weight-based ribavirin (1,000 milligrams or 1,200 milligrams daily) for 48 weeks. Treatment will be stopped at the 12-week mark if the viral level has not fallen 100-fold. Treatment will be stopped at the 24-week mark if the viral level is still detectable.

- Patients with genotype 2 or 3 are usually treated with the standard peginterferon dose and ribavirin 800 milligrams daily for 24 weeks. Some doctors use weight-based ribavirin dosing in patients with genotype 2 or 3.

Your doctor will follow you very closely while you are receiving treatment. It is important that you are honest with your doctor about how you are feeling while on treatment. Blood tests will be performed almost weekly for the first month and then monthly for the rest of treatment. Office visits are scheduled at least monthly.

Robert's comments:

I was diagnosed with genotype 2, which was good news at the time because it responds to treatment much better than type 1 and it requires 24 weeks of treatment as opposed to 48 weeks with type 1. At week 4 of treatment, I had a negative viral load level, which was better news. Again at week 12, I was negative. My doctor discussed the possibility of stopping treatment at this point, citing the study mentioned here. He explained that the study involved patients on a higher dose of ribavirin than I was on, so it was not an exact comparison for me. Because my side effects at this time were getting better, and because if I did relapse later I would have to restart treatment from the beginning, I decided to continue. If you are faced with a decision like this, make sure you know your thyroid condition as well as your white and red blood cell counts, as this information will influence your decision. Your doctor must advise you as to the pros and cons of this situation, but the final decision is yours.

44. What is my chance of being cured?

The approximate cure rates are a 50 percent overall cure rate, a 40 to 45 percent cure rate in patients with genotype 1, and a 70 to 80 percent cure rate in patients with genotypes 2 and 3.

This question can be answered in many different ways depending on how specifically a patient is characterized. The approximate cure rates are a 50 percent overall cure rate, a 40 to 45 percent cure rate in patients with genotype 1, and a 70 to 80 percent cure rate in patients with genotypes 2 and 3. Most of these numbers were derived from three large studies published between 2001 and 2004. Because these studies did not use the same treatment protocols, it is hard to compare their results directly. All three studies compared the combination of a then-new peginterferon in combination with ribavirin to standard interferon and ribavirin.

In 2001, Manns and colleagues published a study comparing the safety and efficacy of two different regimens of peginterferon alfa-2b (Peg-Intron) in combination with ribavirin compared with standard interferon alfa-2b plus ribavirin. The high-dose Peg-Intron group had the best cure rates. This group received the now-standard Peg-Intron dose of 1.5 micrograms per kilogram but only 800 milligrams daily of ribavirin. The overall cure rate was 54 percent. Genotype 1 patients had a cure rate of 42 percent, and genotype 2 and 3 patients had a cure rate of 82 percent. We would expect a higher cure rate in the genotype 1 patients if a higher ribavirin dose had been used, and a review of the data correcting for weight supported this expectation.

In 2002, Fried and colleagues published a study comparing the efficacy and safety of peginterferon alfa-2a (Pegasys) plus ribavirin, standard interferon alfa-2b plus ribavirin, and peginterferon alfa-2a and placebo. In this study, the dose of ribavirin was based on the patient's weight, as is now standard practice in genotype 1 patients. The Pegasys dose was the standard 180 micrograms per week. The group that received Pegasys plus ribavirin had the best cure rates. The overall cure rate was 56 percent. Genotype 1 patients had a cure rate of 46 percent, and genotype 2 and 3 patients had a cure rate of 76 percent. Obviously, the results from these two studies were very similar despite differences in dosing of ribavirin and some other more technical differences.

In 2004, Hadziyannis and colleagues published a study in which all patients were treated with Pegasys but the ribavirin dose (800 milligrams daily versus weight-based 1,000–1,200 milligrams daily) and treatment duration (24 versus 48 weeks) were varied. The results of this study support the current treatment guidelines. Genotype 1 patients did better with 48 weeks of treatment and weight-based ribavirin. Genotype 2 and 3 patients did not benefit from longer-duration treatment or higher ribavirin doses.

All three studies concluded that better cure rates can be achieved when treatment discontinuations and dose reductions are minimized. Other factors besides genotype affect the cure rate as well, as we will discuss in the next question. Creating a model that takes into account all of these other factors poses quite a challenge.

45. What factors other than genotype affect my chance of achieving a response to treatment?

Genotype is clearly the most important predictor of a response to combination therapy. The cure rate for genotype 1 patients is approximately 40 to 45 percent, and that for genotype 2 and 3 patients is 70 to 80 percent. Once treatment has been started, the EVR points at 12 and 24 weeks are strong predictors of treatment response. Studies have also shown that response to treatment improves when patients are able to follow the treatment protocol exactly. The "80:80:80 rule" sums up this relationship: Response is better when patients take at least 80 percent of the peginterferon dose and 80 percent of the ribavirin dose 80 percent of the time. Maintaining the planned treatment regimen for the first 12 weeks appears to be especially important. Obviously, following the treatment protocol 100 percent of the time is the best approach. Treatment interruptions and modifications can result from problems with patient adherence or from doctor-initiated changes in therapy because of side effects. This is why patients are screened carefully before starting therapy and followed closely once therapy begins. Other, harder-to-quantify patient factors also influence the overall chance of a cure. The most important of these other factors are patient age, patient race, presence of **immunosuppression** or human immunodeficiency virus coinfection, viral level, and the amount of scarring on the initial liver biopsy. The data on most of these other factors are less well supported, but it does appear that African

Immunosuppression

suppression of the body's immune system; used after transplants to prevent the body's immune system from damaging the transplanted organ.

American patients and patients older than age 60 are harder to treat. It is hoped that future studies will clarify why and exactly how these patient factors affect the overall cure rate. Any type of immunosuppression (such as is found in transplant patients) and HIV coinfection lower the response rate, most likely due to the decrease in the patient's immune function (Table 7). These conditions represent a double handicap to a patient: Not only do they make treatment less effective, but affected patients have a higher chance of disease progression. Studies have repeatedly shown that lower viral levels and less scarring on the initial liver biopsy are associated with improved response rates. Your doctor will assess all of this information when discussing the risks and benefits of treatment.

46. Can I stop treatment once I start?

Treatment for hepatitis C can be stopped at any point. There is no special risk associated with starting treatment and stopping prematurely. Of course, the chance of achieving a cure is highest if treatment is continued at the full dose for the full time period. Patients are monitored very closely once therapy

Table 7 Factors that Determine Response to Treatment
Genotype
Medication Compliance
Age
Race
Immunosuppression
HIV coinfection
Viral level
Amount of scarring on liver biopsy

begins. If side effects become unacceptable, then treatment can be stopped. The usual reasons for stopping therapy include mood disturbances, excessive flu-like symptoms such as fever and muscle aches, and low blood counts. It is important to be honest with your doctor about how you are feeling once therapy begins. Treatment side effects and their management are discussed in depth in Part 6, "Treatment Side Effects."

47. What are the possible outcomes of treatment, and what happens if I am not cured?

After treatment, every patient is classified as a sustained responder, a relapser, a partial responder, or a nonresponder.

Sustained responder: a patient who has an SVR as defined by an undetectable viral level on blood tests performed 6 months after the end of treatment. This outcome is considered a cure. No further treatment is necessary as long as the viral level remains undetectable, which it usually does.

Relapser: a patient who has an undetectable viral level on blood tests performed at the end of treatment but a detectable viral level 6 months later.

Partial responder: a patient who has a significant (100-fold) drop in viral levels but never has an undetectable viral level.

Nonresponder: a patient who has no significant drop in viral levels at any point during treatment.

Sustained responder

a patient who has a sustained virological response (SVR).

Relapser

a patient who has an undetectable viral level on blood tests performed at the end of treatment for hepatitis C, but a detectable viral level when blood tests are performed 6 months later.

Partial responder

a patient who has a significant (100-fold) drop in viral levels, but never achieves an undetectable viral level, during treatment for hepatitis C.

Nonresponder

a patient who does not experience a significant drop in viral levels at any point during his or her treatment for hepatitis C.

Obviously, patients who are nonresponders, partial responders, or relapsers have not successfully cleared the virus and need to reassess their situation. In general, relapsers appear to respond best to more treatment because they were able to at least temporarily achieve an undetectable viral level. There is no standard approach for treating patients who have failed combination therapy. Different doctors may give the same patient very different advice.

It is important to realize that even without complete clearance of virus, treatment of hepatitis C may slow down the disease's progression. Regardless of what happens in the future, if you have tried therapy, you can move forward with the knowledge that you have taken a proactive approach to your disease. We almost always recommend taking a break from treatment before considering alternatives. Unfortunately, there are no great treatment alternatives available at this time. The two major factors when deciding your next step are the extent of liver damage and your ability to tolerate the treatment.

We do not recommend any further treatment in patients who have mild to moderate scarring on the baseline liver biopsy. These individuals are unlikely to progress to cirrhosis quickly (if at all), and the risks of further treatment might well outweigh the potential benefits. These patients should make appropriate lifestyle modifications and receive follow-up care every 6 to 12 months consisting of liver function tests and an office visit to discuss any changes in their condition and any new treatment options. The liver biopsy should be repeated every few years. Although there is no set guideline, most doctors usually recommend an interval of 3 to 5 years between biopsies.

Patients with more advanced disease, including those with cirrhosis, face a more difficult decision. These individuals are at risk for developing liver-related complications within a few years, so they do need to consider alternative treatment options. There are two major mainstream medical options available for these patients, and we will discuss them in more detail in the next two questions. The first option is the use of maintenance peginterferon, in which a low dose of interferon is used indefinitely in an attempt to control (but not cure) the infection. The second option is the use of an interferon product known as consensus interferon. Some patients, especially relapsers, also opt to try another course of standard combination therapy.

Other options for patients who have failed standard therapy include participation in clinical studies and **complementary and alternative medicine** options. Only a small minority of patients are interested in pursuing clinical studies with experimental drugs and protocols. A good starting point if you are interested in this option is the NIH's website (www.-clinicaltrials.gov), which lists active studies.

48. What is the role for maintenance therapy?

Maintenance therapy involves the indefinite use of peginterferon at a lower dose. The rationale is that maintenance peginterferon will control the virus level, which in turn will reduce the amount of inflammation in the liver and stop the progression of fibrosis. Conceptually, maintenance therapy means that we stop thinking of hepatitis C as an infection and approach it the way that we approach chronic illnesses like hyper-

---

Complementary and alternative medicine

alternatives to standard medical treatment that include supplements, relaxation, massage, and prayer.

Maintenance therapy

indefinite use of peginterferon at a lower dose to treat chronic hepatitis C.

tension and diabetes. Blood pressure medicines do not cure hypertension, but rather seek to control hypertension and decrease the risk of complications such as heart attack and stroke. Similarly, maintenance therapy will not cure hepatitis C but by controlling the virus level it may prevent the development of complications such as liver cancer and liver failure.

Currently, two large, multicenter studies are investigating this hypothesis. The Hepatitis C Antiviral Long-Term Treatment against Cirrhosis study is using peginterferon alfa-2a (Pegasys) monotherapy for up to 4 years in patients who have failed standard combination therapy. Only patients who have advanced fibrosis or cirrhosis are eligible for participation in this study. The Colchicine versus Peg-Intron Long-Term (COPILOT) study is using peginterferon alfa-2b (Peg-Intron) at 0.5 microgram per kilogram per week (one-third of the regular dose) in patients with at least stage 3 disease who have failed standard combination therapy. The COPILOT study recently reported 2-year results showing that patients who were treated with Peg-Intron had a significant decrease in the complication of bleeding compared to the control group, which was treated with an oral medicine called colchicine. No decrease in the risk of liver failure, liver cancer, need for liver transplant, or death was found with Peg-Intron maintenance therapy, however. Final results from these studies should be available within a few years.

Maintenance therapy should be considered in patients with advanced fibrosis or compensated cirrhosis who do not respond to standard combination therapy and who tolerate treatment reasonably well. There is no set recommendation on how to follow patients on maintenance therapy. Viral levels should be monitored, and some doctors continue treatment only if the patient's viral level becomes undetectable or is significantly reduced. Maintenance therapy may not offer any significant benefit in patients who do not demonstrate an appropriate viral level drop.

49. What is the role for consensus interferon?

Consensus interferon is a synthetic interferon that was created by sequencing many natural interferons and using the most common amino acid at each position in the molecule. The goal was to create a more potent interferon molecule. Consensus interferon has been studied in combination with ribavirin in patients who have failed combination therapy. Currently, a large multicenter trial is examining the combination of daily consensus interferon with ribavirin. While preliminary results have been encouraging, the combination's side-effect profile is considerably more severe than that found with standard treatment protocols. This approach must be considered experimental until more data become available.

50. Can I choose not to have treatment?

Many patients decide to defer drug treatment after carefully reviewing the risks and benefits of therapy with their doctors. With this "watchful waiting" approach, patients are monitored and their decision to forgo treatment can be reassessed at any point. Watchful waiting, therefore, should involve a careful initial evaluation of the extent of liver damage (usually with a liver biopsy) and an assessment of the safety of treatment. The decision to defer treatment is usually made in situations in which the person has minimal liver damage or where interferon and ribavirin have significant risks in the specific patient.

Watchful waiting does not mean that nothing is done. If you make the decision to delay treatment, you should continue to see your doctor on a regular basis. During these visits, your doctor will reassess your condition and may eventually decide that currently available medicines are now appropriate. You will also have a chance to review any new treatment options that have become available since your last visit. Similar to the management of patients who have failed treatment, a liver biopsy should be repeated every 3 to 5 years and lifestyle modifications should be continued. Many patients will never progress to cirrhosis, and newer, safer medications may become available within the next few years to treat the patients who do show signs of disease progression.

PART SIX

Treatment Side Effects

Are there any treatment side effects?

What are the side effects of interferon therapy?

What are the side effects of ribavirin therapy?

More...

51. Are there any treatment side effects?

Many patients have no symptoms associated with their hepatitis C infection and are asked to start treatments that will probably make them feel significantly sicker than they currently feel and may even have irreversible side effects. Choosing to initiate treatment is a very difficult decision for many patients, and it is important to understand the risks and benefits before starting therapy. Part 5, "Treatment," spent a long time discussing the benefits of therapy. As noted there, maintaining therapy at the recommended dose and for the recommended time period increases a patient's chance of achieving treatment success. Part 6 discusses the risks of therapy and reviews ways to make treatment more tolerable. The goal is to maintain patient safety and to complete the treatment course.

Both interferon and ribavirin have potentially life-threatening complications, and it is important to thoroughly understand their possible side effects before you begin taking them. Your doctor can measure and check many things, but some side effects—including your mood—cannot be measured. For this reason, it is important for you to be honest with your doctor about how you are feeling. The next series of questions will discuss what to do if you develop specific complications, including flu-like symptoms, fatigue, insomnia, depression, digestive problems, anemia, or thyroid disease. Finally, you should understand that sometimes treatment should be stopped.

Robert's comments:

I decided to start treatment on a Friday in November, so I would have the weekend to recuperate before I returned to work on Monday. Also, most of my personal hobbies are in the summer so I thought that if side effects got bad, they would be easier to tolerate in the winter months (New England) than during summer. A good idea is to keep a daily log of how you feel, your sleep patterns, your physical activity, and what you eat. You may be able to see patterns develop that you can connect to your better (or worse) days. Make sure you discuss your upcoming situation with your spouse, parent, or good friend. Explain to them that you may not be yourself and that you may become moody, and ask them for their help during this time. It would have been much harder for me to go through this ordeal without my wife (and her understanding) by my side. Also talk to your boss and colleagues at work and try to make arrangements for missed time. I was lucky, being able to work from home periodically.

Another thing to do is get a baseline eye exam before and after treatment. It will help pinpoint any eye problems that develop.

52. What are the side effects of interferon therapy?

Interferon is a powerful protein that helps the body fight infections. Unfortunately, it has many potential side effects. Most of these side effects are worse at the beginning of treatment and tend to diminish as treatment is continued. Treatment side effects can be divided into common ones (those seen in at least 10 percent of patients in clinical studies) and less common ones:

Common Side Effects

- Flu-like symptoms such as fever, fatigue, muscle aches, and headaches
- Weight loss
- Nausea and vomiting
- Injection-site irritation
- Hair loss (usually reversible)
- Irritability and depression
- Bone marrow suppression

Uncommon Side Effects

- Thyroid disease
- Autoimmune disease
- Severe infection
- Severe bone marrow suppression, including a low white blood count, low hematocrit, or low platelet count
- Seizures
- Severe depression or psychiatric problems
- Eye problems
- Hearing loss

Your doctor will evaluate you prior to starting therapy with all of these potential side effects in mind and will not recommend treatment if he or she feels that the risks outweigh the benefits. Patients should not be treated with interferon if they have uncontrolled depression or psychiatric problems, an active infection, problems with their bone marrow, an uncontrolled autoimmune disease, active substance abuse, the inability to practice birth control, or any other major medical problem that significantly limits expected lifespan. Interferon should not be used in pregnant women. Some patients will develop worsening liver disease while on interferon therapy. It is hard to distinguish whether this complication is directly related to the interferon therapy or the progression of the underlying hepatitis C infection. One concern is that interferon can precipitate a second liver disease called autoimmune hepatitis. If your liver function tests worsen while you are on therapy, your doctor will test you for autoimmune hepatitis by performing blood tests and possibly a biopsy. In some cases, treatment will be stopped.

Obviously, treatment will be stopped if you develop any of the severe side effects of interferon therapy. It is important for you to be honest with your doctor about how you are feeling, especially regarding mood and depression, because this cannot be measured directly. Most of the common side effects can be treated in an attempt to at least lessen their intensity.

Robert's comments:

The day after my first interferon shot, I started feeling flu-like effects. I had a slight temperature (101°F) and all the classic flu symptoms—sensitive skin, some joint pain, hot flushed skin, and fatigue. These got better day by day, and by midweek I felt better. As time went on, the flu-like symptoms and the joint pain diminished. After about 3 months I noticed my hair thinning and, as of this writing (4 weeks after the end of treatment), I have noticed that it seems to be stopping. I tolerated moodiness pretty well, and I'm sure that was due in most part to having understanding loved ones and friends close by.

53. What are the side effects of ribavirin therapy?

Ribavirin is generally better tolerated than interferon but can also have severe side effects. Several specific concerns must be addressed before any patient starts ribavirin therapy, including pregnancy status and birth control, renal function, potential risk for heart attack and stroke, and other medications. Patients should not be treated with ribavirin if they have a severe baseline anemia, kidney dysfunction, heart disease, risk for strokes, or inability to practice adequate birth control.

In animal studies, ribavirin has been shown to cause birth defects; for this reason, it should not be given to women who are pregnant or who are not practicing adequate birth control. Pregnancy should be avoided for a full 6 months after treatment has been stopped. Men on ribavirin should follow the same precautions.

Hemolysis

the destruction of red blood cells.

Ribavirin can cause a severe and sudden anemia through a mechanism called **hemolysis**, in which red blood cells are destroyed. Because ribavirin is excreted by the kidneys, patients with kidney dysfunction can develop even more severe cases of hemolysis. Patients with severe renal dysfunction should not be treated with this medication. The red blood cells carry oxygen, so the sudden development of anemia can lead to a heart attack or a stroke in patients who are at risk for these complications. As a consequence, doctors will not prescribe this medication for patients with known heart disease and will order a stress test for anyone at risk for heart disease before beginning ribavirin.

Ribavirin can also have significant interactions with some of the antiviral medications used to treat human immunodeficiency virus. Other potential side effects include fatigue and irritability, skin rashes, itching, nasal congestion, cough, and shortness of breath. These side effects are usually mild and do not affect therapy, although sometimes the lung symptoms can become severe and lead to a dose reduction or discontinuation. Overall, the addition of ribavirin improves cure rates significantly, but it worsens the side-effect profile of therapy.

Robert's comments:

I seemed to tolerate the interferon better than the ribavirin. My side effects from ribavirin included a persistent cough, dry mouth, and bad breath initially. All of these disappeared after about 2 months. Lack of concentration and memory loss seemed to get worse with time. Of all the side effects, an itchy skin rash bothered me the most. The rash started about 1 month into the treatment and got progressively worse. At its worst state, it affected my arms, shoulders, chest, back, and legs. It resembled and felt like poison ivy.

54. What can I do about sleep problems, fatigue, and flu-like symptoms?

Sleep problems, fatigue, and flu-like symptoms are the most common side effects of hepatitis C therapy and affect most people to some extent. Controlling these symptoms as much as possible will help you deal with the stresses of everyday life, which will obviously continue while you are on therapy.

Sleep problems are commonplace with hepatitis C and can worsen other potential side effects, especially your mood. You can take several steps to help improve your sleep. Develop good sleep habits, including following a regular schedule of when you wake up and when you go to sleep. Continue to maintain all of your lifestyle modifications, including regular exercise, a healthy diet, and alcohol abstinence. Minimize caffeine intake, especially close to bedtime. Naps can be helpful, but try to avoid long daytime naps because they will make it harder to get to sleep at night. One specific change that sometimes helps with sleep problems is to take ribavirin pills in the late afternoon instead of at bedtime—this medicine can make patients feel jittery.

Fatigue is the most common side effect in patients taking combination therapy. Although it is usually a nonspecific side effect, fatigue can sometimes be related to a specific complication such as anemia or thyroid disease. Your doctor will test for these complications on a regular basis. If you feel that your level of fatigue has suddenly changed, however, you should inform your doctor immediately. The general approach to dealing with fatigue is the same as for sleep problems: regular exercise, a healthy diet, naps as needed, and enough sleep. Many patients feel worse for a few days after the interferon shot. During this time, you should make sure that you get enough fluids and ask your doctor whether you can take some over-the-counter (OTC) acetaminophen or ibuprofen. Always check with your doctor before taking any medications (even OTC ones) while you are on therapy.

Flu-like symptoms such as fever and muscle aches are most severe the first few days after the interferon shot but typically disappear by the end of the week before the next shot. These symptoms tend to lessen with each interferon shot as treatment continues. You should drink enough fluids to stay well hydrated, stay active, and carefully use OTC fever and pain medications as prescribed by your doctor. If a fever does not go away after a day or two or if you have specific symptoms that suggest a localized infection, you should see your doctor.

Robert's comments:

I generally slept okay. There were times when I could not sleep. My sleep problems were due to either joint pain or itchy skin. Tylenol PM seemed to help, except when the itch got bad. I tried an assortment of skin ointments and over–the-counter medications like Benadryl. At best, the ointments offered temporary relief. Gold Bond medicated lotion seemed to offer reliable relief. Benadryl also worked well but caused side effects like sleepiness and a general "spacey" feeling. I found that a hot shower followed by a good-quality moisturizing lotion like Eucerin or Aveeno also worked well. At this writing (4 weeks after the end of treatment), I still have some rash, although it is disappearing. The itching, however, is not disappearing as quickly.

55. What can I do about irritability and depression?

Depression and other psychiatric problems are a serious potential complication of interferon. Uncontrolled psychiatric disease is a contraindication to starting interferon. Any patient with a history of psychiatric problems should consider seeing a psychiatrist before starting treatment. In addition, some doctors will request a consult before allowing a patient to start interferon. The purpose of this consult is twofold: to make sure that it is safe to start interferon and to have a psychiatrist available if problems develop while on treatment. Some doctors will start patients on a mild antidepressant prior to starting interferon. Because your doctor cannot perform a blood test for depression, you need to be honest at your visits regarding how you are feeling.

There are some steps you can take if you develop problems with mild anxiety, irritability, or depression on treatment. For mild anxiety and irritability, try relaxation techniques such as yoga or meditation, exercise on a regular schedule, avoid caffeine, and get enough sleep. Talking about how you feel can help, so many patients rely heavily on friends and family or join a support group after beginning hepatitis C therapy. Minimizing the stressors in your life both at home and at work can help—of course, this can be difficult to accomplish. Some patients also find it helpful to remember that irritability and depression are "expected" side effects of therapy.

You should contact your doctor immediately if your anxiety, irritability, or depression increases and you do not feel that you can control your symptoms. Your doctor may prescribe medications, refer you to a psychiatrist, or even stop therapy. It is important to remember that safety comes first. Therapy can be stopped and restarted at a later date once side effects have been dealt with.

Robert's comments:

In hindsight, I know some activity or exercise would have helped me deal with the side effects better. I spent the first 2 months going to the couch whenever I felt fatigued. After a while, I felt so bored that I started doing some small things around the house even when I felt like lying down. This small amount of exercise gradually made me feel much better and was probably the main reason the fatigue effects disappeared.

56. What can I do about digestive problems?

Digestive problems such as loss of appetite, nausea and vomiting, diarrhea, and mouth problems such as dryness, a bad taste, or soreness are very common side effects of hepatitis C therapy. It is important to monitor and relieve these symptoms because they will affect your overall health and ability to tolerate treatment.

A poor appetite can compromise your overall nutritional status, which in turn may significantly reduce your ability to fight infections in general. Some patients find it easier to eat multiple small meals each day as opposed to three large meals. Try to consume a healthy, well-balanced diet that includes an adequate amount of protein and high-quality carbohydrates. If you are unable to maintain your weight, try nutritional supplements such as Ensure or Carnation Instant Breakfast. These supplements are available in many different flavors, and you should find one that appeals to you.

Mouth problems may include a bad taste, dry mouth, or sore mouth. These issues can severely affect your ability to maintain adequate nutrition. If you develop a bad taste in your mouth, try eating tart foods; their tartness can mask the bad taste. You can also eat cold foods, use lozenges and gum, or try rinsing your mouth with tea or salt water before eating. If you develop a dry mouth, drink lots of fluids and stay well hydrated. You can also try moistening your food, sucking candies or chewing gum, and rinsing your mouth. Mouth ulcers and a sore mouth can develop as a reaction to ribavirin and can be terribly uncomfortable. If you experience these problems, try eating soft or pureed foods or drinking nutritional supplements or milkshakes. In severe cases, your doctor can give you a prescription mouthwash that includes the anesthetic lidocaine.

Nausea and vomiting can be side effects of interferon or ribavirin therapy and can lead to dehydration, which will in turn worsen just about every other side effect. Try following the classic BRATT (bananas, rice, applesauce, tea, toast) diet, eating smaller meals, and sipping carbonated beverages. In severe cases, your doctor can prescribe a medication for nausea.

Diarrhea is a less common side effect that should be treated with diet adjustment, fluids, and increased fiber intake. In severe cases, your doctor can recommend OTC or prescription antidiarrheal medications.

Robert's comments:

I generally eat well and did not have any diet issues during the treatment. I would expect, though, a diet prima-

rily of fast food would cause many more problems with fatigue symptoms.

57. What if I develop anemia while on treatment?

Anemia (low red blood cell count) is an almost universal side effect for patients on combination therapy. Mild anemia can be related to a generalized bone marrow suppression from interferon; severe anemia usually is related to hemolysis due to ribavirin. Your doctor will follow you for symptoms of anemia and will monitor your blood count closely while you are on therapy. While anemia can lead to fatigue, the main concern is that a sudden and severe drop in the red blood cell count can lead to a heart attack or stroke in susceptible patients. Your doctor may take any of several actions if you develop anemia, including lowering the dose of ribavirin or stopping the medication completely, lowering the dose of interferon or stopping the medication completely, or adding a medicine called erythropoietin.

Erythropoietin is a hormone produced by the kidneys that stimulates the bone marrow to produce red blood cells. Several companies manufacture this medicine, whose trade names include Epogen, Procrit, and Aranesp. Treatment of anemia with erythropoietin has been shown to allow continuation of higher ribavirin doses and to improve quality of life for patients while on treatment. The assumption is that improved adherance to recommended treatment regimens will lead to better cure rates.

Treatment with erythropoietin has evolved into the standard of care when patients develop a severe anemia. The usual cutoff for starting treatment is a hemoglobin level of 10 grams per deciliter. Your doctor may also temporarily reduce your ribavirin dose until your red blood cell count rises. The following recommendations are supplied by the manufacturers of the peginterferons for patients with no history of heart disease:

- Hemoglobin < 10 grams per deciliter: decrease ribavirin by 200 milligrams per day
- Hemoglobin < 8.5 grams per deciliter: stop both medicines permanently

Your doctor may follow a slightly different approach with patients who develop anemia, so it is important to discuss the rationale for any treatment changes.

58. What if I develop a low white blood cell count while on treatment?

Neutropenia

a low neutrophil (white blood cell) count.

Neutropenia (a low white blood cell [WBC] count) is another common side effect of hepatitis C therapy related mostly to the bone marrow suppression from interferon. WBCs fight infection, so a low WBC count increases a person's risk of developing a serious infection. Serious infections were seen in a small number (2–4 percent) of patients in the initial peginterferon studies. While the WBC count was not clearly related to the development of infection, doctors tend to remain cautious and adjust the interferon dose when the counts fall low enough. In general, the WBC count tends to decline during the first 2 weeks of therapy and then stabilize. The WBC count returns to normal rapidly after treatment ends. In large studies, neutropenia led to dose reduction of peginterferon in about 20 percent of patients but rarely (< 1 percent) required stopping peginterferon therapy altogether.

The drug known as granulocyte colony-stimulating factor stimulates the bone marrow to produce more WBCs. It is used when the WBC count falls low enough—usually < 500 cells/mm^3. In terms of adjusting the peginterferon dose, peginterferon manufacturers have made the following recommendations:

- WBC < 750 cells/mm^3: decrease peginterferon dose (different amount for the two peginterferons)
- WBC < 500 cells/mm^3: stop peginterferon (one manufacturer says permanently; the other says to restart peginterferon at a half-dose when the WBC level reaches 1,000 cells/mm^3)

Similar to the management of anemia, your doctor may have a slightly different approach.

59. What if I develop a low platelet count while on treatment?

Thrombocytopenia (low platelet count) is another potential side effect related to the bone marrow suppression of interferon. Thrombocytopenia poses a slightly different problem than anemia and neutropenia for several reasons: Thrombocytopenia is often seen in patients with cirrhosis, and no effective stimulating factor for platelets is available. This condition is related to enlargement of the spleen; the enlarged spleen filters blood excessively and removes platelets leading to a low platelet count. A low platelet count often prevents treatment of patients with cirrhosis.

Thrombocytopenia
a low platelet count.

Interleukin-11 (IL-11) can stimulate the bone marrow to produce platelets but is not used in this situation. The main reason is that IL-11 can lead to fluid retention, which is already a potential problem in cirrhotics (the major group of patients who would have a low platelet count). The presence of thrombocytopenia in a patient who is not cirrhotic should prompt further evaluation, probably by a hematologist or blood specialist. The danger is that hepatitis C may cause an autoimmune thrombocytopenia, and interferon treatment may worsen this problem.

The two peginterferon manufacturers have slightly different recommendations, but the general consensus is to decrease the interferon dose when the platelet count falls below 50,000 cells/mm^3 and to stop treatment when the platelet count falls below 25,000 cells/mm^3. We rarely start treatment in patients with a platelet count less than 50,000 cells/mm^3; if we initiate therapy, we follow the platelet count very closely.

60. What if I develop thyroid disease while on treatment?

Thyroid problems develop in as many as 5 percent of patients on combination therapy. The thyroid gland is located in the front of the neck and controls many parts of overall metabolism. Thyroid disease can lead to almost any symptom, including fatigue, loss of appetite, weight loss, digestive problems, and difficulty concentrating. Many of these symptoms are routinely seen in patients on combination therapy, so doctors check thyroid levels on a regular basis. Interferon can lead to either an overactive or an underactive thyroid gland, although underactivity is much more common.

Thyroid problems that develop as a result of interferon treatment are often permanent. Luckily, treatment is usually simple, consisting of just one pill per day of thyroid replacement.

61. What are some other, less common side effects?

Other potential side effects of hepatitis C therapy include hair loss, skin rashes, injection-site reactions, shortness of breath, and vision changes.

Hair loss occurs in about 1 of every 3 patients on interferon and can be quite troubling for some patients. The good news is that hair loss is usually slow and reversible after treatment stops.

Skin rashes are a side effect of ribavirin therapy. They typically occur on the torso and arms and tend to come and go. Some patients can develop more severe skin problems that lead to discontinuation of treatment. Topical therapy with moisturizing skin lotions such as Aveeno and low-dose steroids such as hydrocortisone are first-line treatment for rashes. If these measures fail, stronger steroid creams or a dermatology consult are the next step.

Injection-site reactions are common and tend to improve after a few days. Topical hydrocortisone is also useful for relieving these reactions. It is important to change the site of injection because repeated injections into the same area can lead to a more severe local reaction.

Shortness of breath can be related to fatigue, deconditioning, or anemia but can sometimes be a sign of a more serious lung reaction. A chest x-ray is a reasonable first test in patients who complain of excessive shortness of breath.

A type of vision problem called retinopathy is an uncommon but potentially serious complication of interferon therapy. Patients with diabetes and hypertension are at higher risk for developing retinopathy, and a baseline eye exam should be considered in these individuals before hepatitis C treatment is started. Screening is not recommended in average-risk patients. Patients who experience a sudden visual problem after initiating treatment should be sent for an immediate eye exam.

62. When should treatment be stopped?

Treatment for hepatitis C involves a careful and continual assessment of the risks and benefits for the individual patient who is being treated. The goal is to safely treat the patient and to try to maintain full doses of interferon and ribavirin. Excessive or unnecessary dose reductions or breaks will decrease the cure rate and potential benefit of therapy for the patient without necessarily reducing the risk of treatment-related side effects. Patients need to be monitored closely. If side effects develop that make the risks of continued treatment unacceptable, then treatment needs to be stopped. Most side effects, however, can be lessened through the interventions discussed earlier or are acceptable to patients.

The degree of scarring on the baseline liver biopsy is also crucial to the decision to stop treatment. We are more likely to stop treatment in a patient with early-stage disease who develops a severe side effect. As mentioned previously, a patient with mild disease may never develop cirrhosis and is more likely to remain stable without therapy until newer, safer medications become available.

Some side effects, however, definitely require stopping treatment. Depression and psychiatric side effects are the most common reasons for discontinuing treatment. You should be honest with your doctor about your mood and your interpersonal interactions at work and at home while taking therapy. Blood count problems (anemia, neutropenia, and thrombocytopenia) often lead to dose modifications but rarely require complete discontinuation of treatment. The platelet count is potentially the biggest problem because it often starts low in patients with cirrhosis, and no platelet-stimulating medicine is available for this patient population. Severe infections require stopping treatment but therapy can usually be restarted once the infection is under control. Less common reasons for stopping treatment include severe injection-site reactions, pneumonitis, flaring of autoimmune diseases, overwhelming fatigue, severe skin reactions, and worsening liver function. The decision to stop treatment needs to be made by each individual patient with his or her doctor after a careful analysis of the risks and benefits of the specific situation.

Treatment for hepatitis C involves a careful and continual assessment of the risks and benefits for the individual patient who is being treated. The goal is to safely treat the patient and to try to maintain full doses of interferon and ribavirin.

PART SEVEN

Special Situations

What if I have a new case of acute hepatitis C infection?

Is acute hepatitis C treated differently?

What if I have mild kidney disease or even kidney failure?

More...

63. What if I have a new case of acute hepatitis C infection?

Hepatitis C is rarely diagnosed during the acute phase of infection with the virus. Almost all patients with hepatitis C are diagnosed during the chronic phase of infection—often years or decades after they originally acquired the virus. These patients are diagnosed because of screening initiated by their doctor for patient risk factors or abnormal liver function tests. Part 5 discussed the treatment of patients with chronic hepatitis C in detail. Here the focus is on the unique features and treatment decisions in patients who present with a case of new or acute hepatitis C.

Acute hepatitis C is usually diagnosed when a patient presents with an acute hepatitis. Acute hepatitis is defined as the sudden development of liver inflammation with abnormal liver function tests and jaundice. Many types of liver disease, including other viral infections, can present as an acute hepatitis. Hepatitis A and hepatitis B are much more commonly found in this situation and should always be excluded as possible diagnoses. Hepatitis C is a rare cause for acute hepatitis but can occasionally be seen. A specific cause may not be found in some cases of acute hepatitis.

Acute hepatitis C is difficult to diagnose with absolute certainty unless the patient has a baseline negative hepatitis C test, an episode of acute hepatitis, and then a positive hepatitis C test. The usual situation is a case of acute hepatitis followed by testing that reveals the presence of hepatitis C virus (HCV) without a baseline negative hepatitis C study. The pitfall is that liver function tests can fluctuate in chronic hepatitis C and reach fairly high levels; in other words, high liver function test results and a positive hepatitis C test can be seen with chronic hepatitis C. A liver biopsy can be helpful in some situations because a patient with acute hepatitis C should have a lot of inflammation and no scar tissue. It is important to realize that the antibody test for hepatitis C can take a few weeks to turn positive after a person is initially exposed to the virus. A direct test for HCV, such as a polymerase chain reaction assay, should be performed if a case of acute hepatitis C is suspected. Doctors will use all of this information to decide whether a specific case represents acute hepatitis C.

64. Is acute hepatitis C treated differently?

It is important to differentiate acute hepatitis C from chronic hepatitis C because there are many differences in the way treatment is approached and given in the two situations. Patients with acute hepatitis C often clear the virus spontaneously, so they should be watched for a few months before initiating therapy. Some studies suggest that a patient with acute hepatitis C, who has jaundice, is more likely to clear the virus spontaneously then a patient who has only mild symptoms at the time of initial infection. There is no exact guideline as to how long to wait to see if a patient clears the virus spontaneously. Recommendations range from waiting anywhere from 2 to 6 months before starting treatment.

Many questions remain about how to treat a patient with acute hepatitis C, and very few studies provide good information on this topic. Recent studies suggest that these patients respond better to treatment than patients with chronic hepatitis C. Treatment should therefore not be delayed for so long that patients enter the chronic phase, in which cure rates are lower.

One relatively large study from Germany studied 44 patients with acute hepatitis C. These patients started treatment about 3 months after the acquisition of infection and were treated with standard interferon for 24 weeks. They had an incredibly high cure rate—98 percent. Most doctors who treat acute hepatitis C substitute peginterferon for standard interferon, although this approach has never been formally studied. There is no standard recommendation about whether ribavirin should be added to the treatment regimen and about the duration of therapy, other than it should continue for at least 6 months.

The underlying theory supporting early treatment of acute hepatitis C is that interferon is more effective before the virus can establish a chronic infection. The need for early treatment must be balanced against the possibility that a patient will clear the virus on his or her own, however. Several treatment regimens are available once the decision to treat has been made. The good news: Patients with acute hepatitis C generally respond better to treatment than patients with a chronic infection.

65. What if I have mild kidney disease or even kidney failure?

This is an important issue because many patients with hepatitis C also have some type of kidney disease. Hepatitis C can even cause kidney problems through the production of antibodies called cryoglobulins that directly attack the kidneys. This problem sometimes provides the main rationale for treating hepatitis C. Mild kidney dysfunction is very common, especially in patients with risk factors such as hypertension or diabetes. Hepatitis C is the most common liver disease in patients with kidney failure who are receiving hemodialysis. These patients are at risk because many had received blood transfusions before screening for hepatitis C became available and because hemodialysis equipment may have been contaminated with HCV.

Treatment of a patient with kidney problems can be more difficult than treatment of the average hepatitis C patient. If you have kidney disease, it is important that you find a doctor who is comfortable with this problem. Ribavirin needs to be avoided or used very carefully at lower dosages depending on the level of kidney dysfunction. Ribavirin destroys red blood cells (hemolysis), which can lead to anemia. Patients with kidney dysfunction do not metabolize ribavirin as quickly as patients with normal kidney function. As a consequence, ribavirin stays in their bodies longer and can lead to very severe hemolysis and potentially life-threatening complications. Interferon can be used in patients with kidney disease, but its side effects are often more severe and the dose is often reduced.

Treatment of a patient with kidney problems can be more difficult than treatment of the average hepatitis C patient.

Several different approaches are used depending on the patient's precise circumstances. Patients with cryo-globulinemia can usually tolerate standard combination therapy as long as their kidney dysfunction is mild. These patients are sometimes placed on maintenance therapy if a cure is not achieved with standard treatment. Patients with mild kidney disease are treated either with interferon alone or with combination therapy with very close monitoring and often with a lower dose of ribavirin.

Patients with kidney failure on hemodialysis are the most challenging group to treat and have some unique issues. Dialysis patients with severe scarring in the liver can occassionally have normal liver function tests. A liver biopsy is therefore very useful to accurately stage dialysis patients. The risks of a biopsy are slightly higher because of the clotting problems associated with kidney failure. The stage of hepatitis C becomes even more important in patients who are considering a kidney transplant. A biopsy is important to exclude cirrhosis, which might disqualify a patient for a kidney transplant or change the planned surgery to a combined kidney and liver transplant. Finally, hepatitis C cannot be treated after a kidney transplant because giving interferon in this situation can cause the body to reject the transplanted kidney. The usual approach in a kidney transplant candidate is to perform a liver biopsy to stage the disease and to treat with interferon alone prior to the kidney transplant.

66. What if I have HIV and hepatitis C?

Coinfection with hepatitis C and human immunodeficiency virus has emerged as a significant problem in the last few years. Several trends account for the growth in the number of coinfected patients. The biggest change is the improved medical treatment of HIV, which has lengthened the life expectancy of HIV-infected individuals. Another contributing factor is that HIV and HCV share some risk factors for transmission, such as intravenous drug use. Finally, hepatitis C appears to progress faster in patients with HIV infection, often reaching cirrhosis within 10 years in HIV-infected people as opposed to 20 to 30 years in individuals who are not infected with HIV. Some current studies of this problem estimate that up to 25 percent of patients with HIV also have hepatitis C and that 250,000 individuals in the United States currently have both infections.

All HIV patients should be screened for hepatitis C. In this case, a direct test for the virus should be performed in addition to an antibody test. In the setting of HIV coinfection, a patient with hepatitis C may not develop a positive antibody test because of problems with antibody production. Treatment of HIV/HCV-coinfected patients is clearly more complicated than treatment of non-HIV-infected patients and should be handled by doctors who are comfortable with this situation. Both doctor and patient need to very carefully assess the risks and benefits of treatment, including the risk of more rapid progression to cirrhosis, the patient's life expectancy, and the risks of treatment. Treatment side effects are more common in HIV/HCV-coinfected patients, as are drug interactions between ribavirin and HIV medications. In general, patients with well-controlled HIV infection should be carefully assessed and offered treatment with standard combination therapy if the benefits outweigh the risks. Consultation with the doctor prescribing the HIV medications is essential, and often those medicines require adjustment to prevent drug interactions. Patients need to be monitored very closely while on therapy.

67. What if I have hepatitis B and hepatitis C?

The combination of hepatitis B and hepatitis C is surprisingly rare in the United States. The rates of coinfection with hepatitis B and hepatitis C are higher in parts of the world where either one of these infections is endemic. The reason for the relatively small number of HBV/HCV patients in the United States is that the two infections have different risk factors for transmission. Hepatitis C is usually acquired through exposure to contaminated blood, whereas hepatitis B is more likely to be acquired through sexual contact.

To date, few good studies and no large studies have focused on how to treat this combination. Blood tests may suggest which virus is more active and dominant. The treatment regimen should then be adjusted to more effectively treat the dominant infection. If hepatitis C is more active, standard combination therapy can be prescribed because pegylated interferon is also used to treat hepatitis B. If hepatitis B is more active, your doctor may prescribe other medications that have greater activity against hepatitis B.

68. What about hepatitis C in children?

An estimated 240,000 children in the United States have a positive hepatitis C antibody test, 50 to 75 percent of whom have active infection with detectable virus. Currently, the primary route of transmission for children is perinatal (mother-to-child transmission at birth). In the past, blood transfusions were also a common route of viral transmission in children. Children are more likely to spontaneously clear infection than adults.

Children appear to have fewer symptoms, fewer abnormal liver function tests, and a slower rate of scarring in the liver. Liver biopsies, however, do show similar findings in both children and adults, and scarring does progress with greater duration of infection.

The decision to treat a child can be very difficult and requires careful consideration of the risks and benefits. The Food and Drug Administration has approved the use of combination therapy with interferon and ribavirin in children between the ages of 3 and 17. Treatment in children appears to produce similar response rates as those seen in adults. Any child with hepatitis C should be evaluated by a doctor with a special interest and experience with this situation.

Special Situations

PART EIGHT

Complementary and Alternative Medicine Options

What is the role of complementary and alternative medicine options in hepatitis C?

What can you tell me about milk thistle?

What can you tell me about licorice root?

More...

69. What is the role of complementary and alternative medicine options in hepatitis C?

Conventional or allopathic medicine is practiced by holders of Medical Doctor or Doctor of Osteopathy degrees. The conventional treatment for chronic hepatitis C includes alfa interferon and ribavirin. However, this therapy is effective in only about 50 percent of patients. In addition, the side effects—for example, flu-like symptoms, nausea, skin reactions, and depression—are intolerable for many people. Thus, an increasing number of patients with hepatitis C are exploring complementary and alternative medicine (CAM) options. Over the past several years, the range of alternatives to conventional therapy for hepatitis C has increased dramatically. The number of randomized trials of complementary interventions has doubled every 5 years. As many as 40 percent of people with liver disease are believed to have used or currently use some form of CAM. Most take herbal supplements like milk thistle or licorice root. Other patients rely on self-prayer, relaxation, massage, or chiropractic therapies.

Most medical experts on hepatitis C believe that no CAM therapy has been proven effective to date because no large-scale scientific studies of these treatments have been performed.

You may have heard various claims regarding CAM either through direct marketing or from other people with liver disease. Most medical experts on hepatitis C believe that no CAM therapy has been proven effective to date because no large-scale scientific studies of these treatments have been performed. To make an informed choice about CAM, it is important to evaluate the evidence carefully. If you are using supplements or CAM, let your physician know.

70. What can you tell me about milk thistle?

The scientific name for milk thistle is *Silybum marianum*. This plant comes from the aster (similar to daisy) family. It is native to the Mediterranean, but can now be found worldwide. It grows in dry, sunny areas and has red and purple flowers. The active ingredient likely comes from the fruit and is called silymarin. It is available in capsules or in liquid form and is used by herbalists to treat liver and gallbladder disease. Silymarin may also be used as a preventive agent or an antidote for mushroom poisoning.

Those who support the use of milk thistle in hepatitis C claim that it relieves congestion in the liver, spleen, and kidneys. Recent studies also suggest that milk thistle may protect the liver by acting as an **antioxidant** and preventing toxins from injuring liver cells. Milk thistle is generally well tolerated but may sometimes have side effects. Gastrointestinal side effects include nausea, diarrhea, flatulence, bloating, and altered **bowel** habits. Other potential side effects of milk thistle include headache, skin reactions, joint aches, impotence, and allergic reactions. Milk thistle can also interact with antipsychotic medications, phenytoin (used for seizures), aspirin, and halothane (an anesthetic).

Most of the published studies with milk thistle have been done in patients with liver disease in general, not hepatitis C specifically. A recent review concluded that milk thistle had no effect on mortality, improvement in liver function tests, or liver histology (tissue analysis).

Antioxidants

vitamins, minerals, and enzymes that reduce damage to cells by neutralizing free radicals.

Bowel

term used for both the large and small intestines.

71. What can you tell me about licorice root?

The scientific name for the licorice plant is *Glycyrrhiza glabra*. Most licorice is produced in Greece, Turkey, and Asia. The active ingredient is a substance called glycyrrhizin, which is made from the peeled and unpeeled dried root of the licorice plant. In cooking, licorice has long been used for flavoring purposes because of its sweetness. Medically, it has a history of use in Europe and Asia for coughs, ulcer disease, sore throats, and inflamed joints.

Studies conducted to date have not produced definitive conclusions about the efficacy of licorice root in hepatitis C. Its mechanism of action is unclear, but it may have antiviral properties that prevent progression to liver cancer in hepatitis C. It may also lower liver function test results. Common side effects include high blood pressure, sluggishness, water retention that produces leg swelling, and headache. Other potential side effects include muscle pain, numbness in the arms and legs, and weight gain. Licorice root can also interact with certain drugs such as diuretics, digoxin, steroids, insulin, oral contraceptives, and heart rhythm medications.

72. What can you tell me about ginseng?

Ginseng belongs to the genus *Panax*. Two different species of ginseng are used as medical herbs: *Panax ginseng* (Asian ginseng) and *Panax quinquefolis* (American ginseng). Ginseng, which comes from a tan root, is claimed to improve mental performance, control blood sugar in adult-onset diabetes mellitus, reduce the risk of various cancers, improve pulmonary function in chronic obstructive lung disease, reduce coronary artery disease, improve exercise performance, enhance the immune system, and reduce menopausal symptoms. In particular, some animal studies have demonstrated that ginseng may increase the ability to resist disease. It is well tolerated by most patients and severe side effects are rare. Potential but mild side effects include skin rash, itching, diarrhea, sore throat, decreased appetite, depression, anxiety, insomnia, and bleeding.

73. What can you tell me about thymus extract?

The thymus is a gland located in the lower part of the neck that is necessary for proper development of the immune system, especially in infants and young children. It produces white blood cells called T lymphocytes, which are important in fighting infection by bacteria, viruses, fungi, yeast, and parasites. The thymus also produces hormones that regulate many immune functions.

Thymus extract, which is usually prepared from calves' thymus glands, works by stimulating the immune system. Potential benefits include improving the function of T lymphocytes in patients with HIV, restoring white blood cells in patients with cancer, relieving asthma, improving symptoms of allergies, and preventing upper respiratory infections such as pneumonia, bronchitis, and sinusitis. Thymus extract may also help patients with acute or chronic hepatitis by improving the immune system, although only small studies have been performed to examine these purported benefits.

This dietary supplement comes as an oral tablet or a capsule. It is not yet available in the United States. There are no known side effects. However, because this supplement comes from cows, there is a theoretical concern that it could transmit infections from cows to humans.

74. What can you tell me about Schisandra?

Schisandra's name in Chinese is *wu-wei-zi*, roughly translated as "five tastes of fruit." This name reflects its varying effects on the palate: sour, sweet, hot, salty, and bitter. There are two species of interest as herbal supplements, both of which are found in China and Russia: *Schisandra chinesis* and *Schisandra sphenanthera*. The fruit, which is the most important part of the plant, grows on vines as red berries.

Some claims have been made that *Schisandra* could be useful for patients with kidney and lung disease. To date, there are no reports of formal studies on the safety and effectiveness of using *Schisandra* alone for treatment of hepatitis C in humans, but this supplement may have a liver-protective effect by acting as an antioxidant. Potential side effects include heartburn, poor appetite, skin rashes, and abdominal pain.

75. What can you tell me about colloidal silver?

Silver has many uses ranging from jewelry to electronics; it has also been used for many years to treat various medical conditions. Today, physicians use silver solutions to treat certain eye infections, skin abnormalities, and burns. Colloidal silver, which consists of tiny silver particles suspended in liquid, is classified as an oral nutritional supplement. The actual amount of silver in each supplement varies depending on its manufacturer.

Colloidal silver may have antimicrobial activities, killing microorganisms such as viruses, bacteria, and fungi. Some people claim that it reduces the occurrence of colds and the flu. So far, scientific studies have not proven any benefit for colloidal silver. In 1999, the Food and Drug Administration stated that products containing silver colloid were not safe or effective in their claims. In fact, the long-term ingestion of this substance may lead to a condition called argyria, in which the skin turns blue-gray; this change may not be treatable or reversible. Colloidal silver may also build up in the internal organs and in the nails. Other potential side effects include headaches, kidney dysfunction, abdominal pain, and malaise. This supplement may also interact with certain antibiotics.

76. What can you tell me about antioxidants?

The food we eat is processed into energy in the body. During these chemical reactions, substances called free radicals are produced. These free radicals may cause signs of aging and contribute to a variety of diseases. Antioxidants are vitamins, minerals, and enzymes that reduce the free radicals' damage to cells and to the deoxyribonucleic acid (DNA) within the cells. Antioxidants in the form of nutritional supplements may also have a similar result.

Vitamin A (which is also known as retinol) is found in many dark green, yellow, and orange vegetables such as carrots, squash, broccoli, tomatoes, kale, and collards. Fruits rich in this antioxidant include cantaloupes, peaches, and apricots. Vitamin C (which is also known as ascorbic acid) is found in fruits such as oranges, limes, lemons, and strawberries. Vegetables rich in ascorbic acid include tomatoes, green peppers, broccoli, cabbage, and green leafy vegetables. Vitamin E is found in nuts, seeds, whole grains, wheat germ, and green leafy vegetables. Selenium and fish oils are other types of antioxidants.

Health claims for antioxidants include that they decrease heart disease, improve diabetes, improve macular degeneration, and prevent chronic diseases. These substances may also protect the liver from damage caused by free radicals. Vitamin E has been demonstrated in one small study to possibly help patients with non-alcoholic steatohepatitis.

77. What can you tell me about zinc?

Zinc is needed to produce the building blocks of the body—DNA and ribonucleic acid. This element is also important in making enzymes and enhancing the function of the immune function. Zinc deficiency can cause growth retardation, delayed sexual maturation, impotence, baldness, skin rash, and impaired taste. Zinc deficiency is common in people living in poor countries, alcoholics, individuals with sickle cell anemia, and people with chronic kidney disease. Zinc excess can cause abdominal pain, diarrhea, nausea, and vomiting. Foods rich in zinc include red meats, shellfish, and whole-grain cereals.

Zinc may enhance the response to interferon therapy in patients with chronic hepatitis C. It may also improve **encephalopathy** (confusion) in those patients with severe liver disease. Zinc may also reduce the duration of colds in adults and improve health in malnourished individuals.

78. What can you tell me about oxymatrine?

The scientific name for oxymatrine is *Sophora*. Approximately 45 different species exist, and the active ingredient can be isolated from their roots. Oxymatrine has long been used in traditional Chinese herbal medicine and as a treatment for cancer, heart abnormalities, skin diseases, and liver disease. Some studies suggest that it may have a protective effect on the liver. Further studies are necessary to prove the effectiveness of oxymatrine more definitively. Possible serious side effects of this supplement include neurologic deficits, movement disorders, and convulsions.

79. What can you tell me about diet?

Patients with hepatitis C should maintain a healthy diet for many reasons. A patient's diet should include enough protein to fight infections and ensure liver regeneration. Hepatitis C patients should consume lots of fruits and vegetables for their antioxidant effects. They should also avoid alcohol and other potentially harmful drugs and toxins. In addition, patients should limit their consumption of high-fat and high-sugar foods and consume plenty of fluids.

Although consuming a healthy diet may not directly affect the hepatitis C virus, it will improve other aspects of a patient's health. Obesity itself can lead to inflammation and scarring in the liver. Diet is especially important for patients who are undergoing treatment for hepatitis C.

PART NINE

Cirrhosis

What is cirrhosis?

How is cirrhosis diagnosed?

What are the signs and symptoms of cirrhosis?

More . . .

80. What is cirrhosis?

The liver is the largest organ in the body, and its proper functioning is essential for survival. The liver's many jobs include clearing the blood of toxins, breaking down old red blood cells, creating clotting factors to control bleeding, producing proteins for nutrition, and creating bile to absorb fats and certain vitamins. Cirrhosis is the pathologic condition in which normal liver tissue is replaced by abnormal fibrous scar tissue. This scarring process prevents the liver from functioning properly and makes it harder for blood to flow through the liver. Because the liver is such an essential organ, its failure creates problems throughout the body.

Cirrhosis is the pathologic condition in which normal liver tissue is replaced by abnormal fibrous scar tissue.

Cirrhosis is the end result of many different chronic liver diseases. The complications associated with cirrhosis are the same regardless of the cause of a patient's liver disease. Cirrhosis kills about 27,000 people per year in the United States, making it the twelfth leading cause of death by disease.

Hepatitis C is the second most common cause of cirrhosis in the United States, after alcoholism. Approximately 20 percent of patients with hepatitis C develop cirrhosis over a period of 20 to 40 years. A patient with hepatitis C and cirrhosis is at risk for developing liver failure and liver cancer. Patients who have hepatitis C and drink alcohol have an even higher risk of developing cirrhosis. Other factors that may influence the progression to cirrhosis include increased age, male gender, coinfection with human immunodeficiency virus, and the presence of fat in the liver.

Because other chronic liver diseases can lead to cirrhosis, patients with hepatitis C are usually screened for most of these other conditions. As mentioned earlier, the most common cause of cirrhosis in the United States is excessive consumption of alcohol. Alcoholic cirrhosis often occurs in patients who consume more than four drinks per day for more than 10 years. Approximately 10 to 15 percent of people who drink alcohol at this level and for this length of time will develop cirrhosis. Hepatitis B and D are other chronic viral diseases that can progress to cirrhosis. In fact, hepatitis B is the most common cause of cirrhosis worldwide. Autoimmune hepatitis is a disease in which the immune system attacks the liver, producing inflammation and eventually scarring. In addition, several inherited liver diseases can cause cirrhosis. Hemochromatosis is a genetic disorder in which iron is inappropriately stored in various organs. In addition to affecting the liver, hemochromatosis can cause fatigue, diabetes, heart failure, arthritis, and various endocrine abnormalities. Other inherited diseases that can cause cirrhosis include alpha-1 antitrypsin deficiency, **Wilson's disease**, and glycogen storage diseases. Finally, chronic diseases of the bile ducts, drugs or toxins, and fatty liver may progress to cirrhosis.

Because the liver interacts with so many other organs, its failure affects the body in numerous ways. The increased pressure in the liver makes it hard for blood to flow through the liver and leads to a condition called **portal hypertension**. Portal hypertension, in turn, can lead to **varices**, hemorrhoids, an enlarged spleen, and a low platelet count. The loss of functioning of the liver can also cause ascites, **spontaneous**

Wilson's disease

a liver disease characterized by abnormal retention of copper in the body.

Portal hypertension

an abnormal increase in pressure within the portal system that usually develops in the setting of cirrhosis.

Varices

dilated veins that are often found in the setting of advanced liver disease. They often occur in the esophagus and stomach and can rupture and bleed.

Spontaneous bacterial peritonitis

infection of ascites; it can be treated with antibiotics.

bacterial peritonitis, and encephalopathy. Patients with cirrhosis are at an increased risk for developing liver cancer. This risk is higher in certain liver diseases, including viral infections such as hepatitis C.

A patient with cirrhosis who has not experienced any major complication and still has reasonably good liver function is said to have compensated cirrhosis. Many people with compensated cirrhosis lead normal lives and visit their doctors twice a year for a checkup, blood tests, and an ultrasound to make sure that nothing has changed. Most patients with hepatitis C and cirrhosis have compensated disease. Patients with cirrhosis who have had any of the major complications associated with this condition are said to have decompensated cirrhosis. These individuals need active medical care, and many are being evaluated for a liver transplant.

81. How is cirrhosis diagnosed?

Cirrhosis is a pathologic diagnosis—in other words, the definitive way to make the diagnosis is to obtain a piece of the liver through a liver biopsy. The small piece of tissue is then examined under the microscope. The amount of scarring is given a score between 0 and 4, where 0 means normal and 4 means cirrhosis. The biopsy sample is also examined for clues about the cause of a patient's liver disease. This cause can usually be determined with a careful history and blood tests before a biopsy, but occasionally a biopsy will help to clarify matters in a confusing case.

A standard liver biopsy is performed percutaneously—that is, the needle is passed through the abdominal wall into the liver. This approach is sometimes impossible in a patient with cirrhosis. An alternative approach that can be used is a **transjugular** biopsy, in which the needle is passed through a neck vein and into the liver via blood vessels.

A liver biopsy is not always necessary in a suspected case of cirrhosis. A doctor who observes certain symptoms, physical exam findings, or abnormal test results may make the diagnosis of cirrhosis without a biopsy. Imaging studies such as ultrasounds, computed tomography (CT) scans, and magnetic resonance imaging (MRI) scans are very useful in this situation as well. A cirrhotic liver often appears nodular and shrunken in these studies. Imaging studies can also show other findings such as ascites, an enlarged spleen, and dilated veins that are strongly suggestive of cirrhosis. A doctor may decide that the diagnosis is so likely that the risk of a liver biopsy outweighs its benefit.

Transjugular
using the internal jugular (IJ) vein within the neck to access different internal structures. The IJ is used during a transjugular intrahepatic portosystemic shunt (TIPS) procedure and occasionally during a liver biopsy.

82. What are the signs and symptoms of cirrhosis?

Patients with cirrhosis can present with a variety of signs and symptoms, ranging from almost nothing to a life-threatening complication. Some patients present with no symptoms, but the diagnosis is made because of a finding such as abnormal liver function tests or an enlarged spleen. Other patients present with relatively minor, nonspecific symptoms such as abdominal pain, exhaustion, fatigue, decreased appetite, and nausea.

More specific symptoms include itching, easy bleeding and bruising, jaundice, and skin changes:

- Cirrhosis can cause blockage of the small bile ducts in the liver, which can lead to a buildup of toxins. These toxins sometimes cause a severe itching sensation.
- The liver produces a large number of proteins that are necessary for blood to clot properly. Cirrhotic patients may produce inadequate amounts of these proteins, and develop excessive bleeding or easy bruising.
- Patients can develop jaundice or yellowing of the skin and eyes. The liver breaks down old red blood cells into bile, which is excreted out of the liver by the bile ducts. These end products of blood are processed more slowly by a cirrhotic liver and can result in yellowing of the skin and eyes when they accumulate.
- Skin changes include redness of the palms (**palmar erythema**) and fine blood vessels on chest and back (**spider telangiectasias**).

Patients with cirrhosis can present with a variety of signs and symptoms, ranging from almost nothing to a life-threatening complication.

Palmar erythema

redness of the palms; it occurs in cirrhosis.

Spider telangiectasias

fine blood vessels on the chest and back that occur in patients with cirrhosis.

83. What are the complications of cirrhosis?

Patients with cirrhosis can develop several major complications including ascites, spontaneous bacterial peritonitis, encephalopathy, bleeding varices, kidney problems, lung problems, and liver cancer. Liver cancer is discussed in detail in Part 10 of this book. This question defines and discusses the other major complications, including treatment options.

Ascites is the abnormal accumulation of fluid in the abdominal cavity. Cirrhosis is a common cause of ascites but not the only one—heart failure, kidney disease, certain cancers, and some infections may also lead to ascites. Some patients have more than one of these conditions. In particular, patients often develop ascites related to both cirrhosis and kidney disease.

The presence of ascites is obvious in many patients, who develop significant abdominal distention or swelling as a result of the fluid buildup. In other cases, ascites may be less obvious and is detected by an imaging study such as an ultrasound or CT scan. Control of ascites initially focuses on diet and medical therapy. Doctors usually recommend that patients with ascites limit their intake of sodium to no more than 2 grams per day. In addition, a patient may be asked to restrict fluid intake. In the absence of kidney dysfunction, ascites is initially treated with diuretics. The two most commonly used diuretic medications are spirinolactone and furosemide. It may take as long as a week for these medications to start working, and blood tests will be performed before your doctor adjusts the dose. Patients with ascites should completely avoid aspirin, ibuprofen, and other **nonsteroidal anti-inflammatory drugs** because they may be harmful to the kidneys.

Refractory ascites refers to abdominal fluid that persists despite diet modification and diuretic therapy. This condition may be treated with a paracentesis every few weeks, a **transjugular intrahepatic portosystemic shunt (TIPS)** procedure, or liver transplantation. A paracentesis is a procedure in which fluid in the abdomen is drained with a needle. In a diagnostic paracentesis, a small amount of fluid is removed for testing; in a therapeutic paracentesis, a large amount of fluid is removed for comfort or to help with breathing.

Nonsteroidal anti-inflammatory drug

a drug such as aspirin or ibuprofen that has both analgesic and anti-inflammatory properties.

Transjugular intrahepatic portosystemic shunt (TIPS)

placement of a stent within the liver to allow increased blood flow through the liver. This procedure can be used to treat ascites or bleeding from varices.

If you have a paracentesis, this is what you may expect. The procedure is performed either as an inpatient or an outpatient procedure in a hospital or a doctor's office. The total time depends on the amount of fluid to be removed but typically takes 15 to 45 minutes to complete. First, the patient is asked to lie down, with the head of the bed being elevated. The procedure is performed using "sterile technique" to reduce the risk of infection. An area in the lower portion of the right or left abdomen is chosen for the site of fluid removal. This area is cleaned thoroughly and drapes are placed over the abdomen. Initially, a small needle is used to provide a local anesthetic or numbing medication. A larger needle is then used to remove the fluid. Occasionally, a radiologist uses and ultrasound probe to locate the ascites and marks skin with ink. If a large amount of ascites is present, several liters of fluid may be removed at one time. If more than 5 liters of fluid are removed, our practice is to give another fluid called albumin through an intravenous (IV) line to reduce the risk of low blood pressure and kidney dysfunction.

Another option for patients with refractory ascites is a TIPS procedure. This procedure involves the placement of a stent into the liver. This stent (or shunt) allows blood to flow more easily through the liver and can help some patients with ascites. The TIPS procedure is also used for patients who have bleeding varices. The final—and best—option for patients with refractory ascites is a liver transplantation.

Infection of ascites is very common because the fluid is attractive to bacteria. Spontaneous bacterial peritonitis

(SBP) is the medical term for the situation in which ascites becomes infected. The term "spontaneous" is used because the infection develops without a clear cause. In contrast, in secondary **peritonitis**, an infection in the abdomen (peritonitis) results from a discrete event such as a perforated ulcer or diverticulitis. The classical presentation of SBP features severe abdominal pain and fever. Some patients can present with milder symptoms, and doctors are always concerned about the possibility of SBP in any patient with ascites who develops a new problem or whose condition changes. In this situation, a paracentesis is performed to rule out an infection. A small amount of fluid is removed during the paracentesis and then sent to the lab. Within a few hours, the lab can usually determine whether an infection is present. If so, antibiotics are indicated for a total of 10 to 14 days. After full treatment, an antibiotic is given to prevent future episodes of SBP. Antibiotics such as ciprofloxacin, levofloxacin, and trimethoprim-sulfamethoxazole are frequently prescribed in this scenario.

Peritonitis
inflammation of the lining that surrounds organs in the abdominal cavity.

Portal systemic encephalopathy (PSE) is another potential complication of cirrhosis. One of the major functions of the liver is to detoxify the blood. In cirrhosis, the liver may become overwhelmed and be unable to remove all of the toxins. Patients may then develop symptoms of PSE, which can range from a mild personality change to confusion to coma. Precipitants of PSE include gastrointestinal bleeding, infection, dehydration, constipation, and use of sedatives. The initial treatment for PSE includes correcting or treating the original cause and use of a medication called lactulose. Lactulose causes loose stools that

Portal systemic encephalopathy (PSE)
confusion and mental status changes that occur in patients with advanced liver disease, most likely due to an increase in abnormal toxins.

reduce the amount of toxins that is absorbed from the intestines. Patients often need to take lactulose every day to prevent PSE. Side effects of lactulose include abdominal cramps, bloating, and diarrhea. Sometimes an antibiotic may be used if lactulose does not work or is poorly tolerated. Neomycin and rifaximin are the most commonly used antibiotics in this situation.

Many patients with cirrhosis develp portal hypertension which means that the blood pressure in the portal vein becomes elevated. This blood vessel drains a large amount of blood from the abdomen into the liver, which then drains into the heart; collectively, this network is known as the **portal system**. Portal hypertension can lead to an enlarged spleen, a low platelet count, and the formation of varices. The portal vein normally has a low pressure; scarring in the liver, however, can increase this pressure. One of the blood vessels that feeds the portal vein is the splenic vein, which drains the spleen. The spleen has several functions including filtering the blood. Portal hypertension can lead to an engorged spleen which can result in excessive filtering of the blood and a low blood platelet level.

Portal system

includes all veins that drain the small and large intestines, stomach, and spleen and that converge into the portal vein to drain into the liver.

The major complication of portal hypertension is the formation of varices—that is, dilated blood vessels. Blood always needs to return to the heart, and it will find other ways back to the heart that bypass the liver. As a consequence, blood vessels that are normally small can become engorged. Occasionally, a blood vessel will become so large that it bursts. In this situation, a patient can develop life-threatening bleeding. The most common locations for bleeding varices are in the **esophagus** and the stomach. An esophageal variceal or gastric variceal bleed is a major complication associated with a 30 percent chance of death.

Esophagus

the muscular tube that carries food from the mouth to the stomach.

Doctors initially treat variceal bleeding with a procedure called an upper endoscopy or an **esophagogastroduodenoscopy (EGD)**. An **endoscope** is a very thin, flexible tube that contains a camera, a light, and an instrument channel. The EGD visualizes the esophagus, the stomach, and a portion of the small intestine. The next question discusses the upper endoscopy procedure in more detail.

Doctors can stop bleeding from varices either by injecting them with a solution that makes the blood clot or by putting a rubber band around the area that is bleeding; a procedure called endoscopic variceaal ligation. Endoscopy with treatment of the varices is repeated on a regular basis until the varices are destroyed completely. Other options for treating a variceal bleed include a TIPS procedure and a surgical shunt called a distal splenorenal shunt.

Many other major complications of cirrhosis are possible, but a full discussion of them is beyond the scope of this book. We will briefly mention some of the kidney and lung problems that can develop as a consequence of cirrhosis. As mentioned earlier, the kidneys are very susceptible to dysfunction in patients with liver disease. Kidney dysfunction progresses in several well-characterized stages. The first stage is an inability to properly excrete sodium from the body; this stage is seen in patients with ascites. The next stage is an inability to properly remove water from the body; this stage is seen in patients with refractory ascites. The third and final stage is when the kidneys fail completely. This condition, which is called **hepatorenal syndrome**, has a very high mortality.

Three major lung problems are observed in cirrhotic patients:

Esophagogastro-duodenoscopy (EGD)

a procedure in which the esophagus, stomach, and duodenum are visualized with an endoscope.

Endoscope

thin, flexible tube with an attached light that is used to view the digestive tract.

Endoscopic variceal ligation

a procedure using small rubber bands to treat varices in the esophagus and stomach.

Hepatorenal syndrome

a type of kidney failure that occurs in the setting of advanced liver disease.

Hepatic hydrothorax

the accumulation of fluid in the lining of the lungs due to liver disease.

Hepatopulmonary syndrome

low oxygen levels in the body due to shunting of blood in the lungs that occurs in the setting of cirrhosis.

Portopulmonary hypertension

high pressures in the blood vessels that enter the lungs in the setting of cirrhosis.

- **Hepatic hydrothorax** is the accumulation of fluid in the lining of the lung. This condition, which is related to ascites, develops when small tears in the diaphragm allow fluid to track up into the lungs.
- **Hepatopulmonary syndrome** is characterized by the shunting of blood through the lungs and a low oxygen level.
- **Portopulmonary hypertension** is a condition in which patients develop high blood pressure in the blood vessels entering the lungs.

All three of these lung problems are serious and are associated with high patient mortality.

84. What should I do if I have cirrhosis?

When a patient receives a diagnosis of cirrhosis, several steps are taken. The first step is to figure out the cause and treat the underlying liver disease if possible. A patient with hepatitis C should be offered treatment if he or she is not too sick. In addition, any complication of cirrhosis should be identified and treated. A patient should institute lifestyle modifications, including alcohol abstinence, diet modification, and appropriate exercise. Medications should be used carefully and checked for potential damage to the liver. Finally, any patient with cirrhosis should have certain screening tests done—namely, screening for liver cancer, varices, and immunity to hepatitis A and hepatitis B.

Hepatoma

cancer of the liver that often occurs in the setting of cirrhosis. Also known as hepatocellular carcinoma.

Hepatocellular carcinoma or **hepatoma** is the fifth most common cancer worldwide. A patient with hepatitis C and cirrhosis has an approximately 2 to 6 percent yearly risk of developing a hepatoma. For this reason, any patient with hepatitis C and documented cirrhosis should be screened for liver cancer on a regular basis. Screening tests may include blood tests such as an **alpha-fetoprotein** level and imaging studies such an ultrasound, a CT scan, or an MRI scan. The rationale for screening is that this type of cancer is more likely to be curable if it is detected at an early stage. A patient who presents with symptoms such as abdominal pain, weight loss, or jaundice is unlikely to have curable disease. Part 10, "Liver Cancer," discusses these issues in more depth.

A patient with cirrhosis is at risk for the development of varices in the esophagus and stomach. Therefore, when a person is first diagnosed with cirrhosis, an upper endoscopy is performed to assess for esophageal or gastric varices. If no varices are seen, this test is repeated every two years. If small varices are seen, the test is repeated every year. If large varices are seen but have not yet begun bleeding, a medication is started to prevent bleeding. The goal is to reduce the pressure in the blood vessels that supply the liver, thereby reducing the risk of bleeding. The medications prescribed for this purpose belong to a class of drugs called nonselective beta blockers; examples include propranolol and nadolol. The doses of these medications are adjusted based on the heart rate. Potential side effects include fatigue, lightheadedness, cold extremities, or exacerbation of asthma.

If nonselective beta blockers are contraindicated, an endoscopy may be recommended to obliterate the varices. This is what you may expect from an upper endoscopy. You will be asked to fast for at least 6 hours before the test so that the stomach is empty and a thorough exam can be completed. Immediately before

Alpha-fetoprotein
a blood test that is often elevated in patients who have liver cancer.

Cirrhosis

the procedure, an IV line is placed, and oxygen is given through your nose. The lights in the room are dimmed, and you are turned on your left side. Often, a topical anesthetic or numbing medication is sprayed into the back of your throat to dull the sensation. Medications are infused through the IV line; these medications cause relaxation and help you forget the procedure. A guard is put in your mouth to protect your gums and teeth. After you are sedated, the endoscope enters your mouth, esophagus, stomach, and first portion of your intestine called the duodenum. The procedure usually takes no more than 5 to 10 minutes, although it may take longer if it includes therapy. Afterwards, you will feel drowsy and lethargic. Many patients do not remember the procedure even happening. It is not safe for you to drive yourself home after an upper endoscopy, so you must come with a family member or friend who does the driving.

As mentioned earlier, current practice is to screen all patients who are diagnosed with hepatitis C for both hepatitis A and hepatitis B. Hepatitis A and hepatitis B are potentially more dangerous in a patient with hepatitis C than in a patient without liver disease. A patient with hepatitis C already has a poorly functioning liver and sometimes cannot tolerate another attack on the liver. One study from Italy showed a high death rate from acute hepatitis A in this situation, even though hepatitis A is otherwise usually self-limited. Many patients have a natural immunity to hepatitis A and do not need vaccination. Anyone who is not immune to hepatitis A or hepatitis B should be vaccinated (Table 8).

Table 8 Complications of Cirrhosis
Ascites
Spontaneous bacterial peritonitis
Encephalopathy
Bleeding varices
Kidney disease
Lung disease
Liver cancer

Cirrhosis

85. Can I be treated for hepatitis C if I have cirrhosis?

Hepatitis C can be treated in patients who have compensated cirrhosis. Patients with decompensated cirrhosis, by contrast, are almost always too sick to tolerate treatment. Some transplant centers have explored the possibility of treating decompensated patients prior to liver transplant in an effort to prevent recurrent hepatitis C after transplantation. This approach is controversial and obviously will be attempted only by experienced hepatologists in transplant centers. In standard practice, only patients with compensated cirrhosis are offered treatment.

A patient with compensated cirrhosis has much to gain from the treatment and cure of hepatitis C. These patients are at risk for liver failure and liver cancer, with the risk being estimated about 5 percent per year. Cure of hepatitis C in this situation offers two major benefits for a patient. First, it reduces the patient's yearly risk of a major complication from 5 percent to 2 percent. Second, if the patient ever needs a liver transplant, the risk of recurrent hepatitis C after transplant

Hepatitis C can be treated in patients who have compensated cirrhosis. Patients with decompensated cirrhosis, by contrast, are almost always too sick to tolerate treatment.

is significantly reduced. This is a major issue because post-transplant hepatitis C has a more aggressive course, with 25 percent of patients developing cirrhosis within 5 years. Treatment of patients with cirrhosis also carries higher risks than treatment of patients in the pre-cirrhotic stage. A cirrhotic patient has fewer reserves to deal with complications, and any worsening of liver function can transform compensated cirrhosis into decompensated cirrhosis. These patients should be followed closely while on treatment.

In summary, patients with compensated cirrhosis should be considered for treatment. Treatment has more potential risks and benefits in these individuals, however, than in pre-cirrhotic patients.

PART TEN

Liver Cancer

Can you give me an overview of liver cancer and hepatitis C?

What are the signs and symptoms of liver cancer?

Who should be screened for liver cancer and how?

More...

86. Can you give me an overview of liver cancer and hepatitis C?

Liver cancer is a common and life-threatening complication in patients with hepatitis C. Many different types of cancers may involve the liver. The broadest distinction is whether the cancer started in the liver (primary cancer) or whether it started in another part of the body and then spread to the liver (metastatic or secondary cancer). Several types of primary liver cancer are distinguished depending on what type of liver cell becomes cancerous. Patients with hepatitis C almost always develop a type of primary liver cancer called hepatocellular carcinoma (hepatoma, for short). Hepatoma is the most common form of liver cancer in adults and is the focus of the discussion in this book.

There are also a variety of benign liver tumors that can be hard to distinguish from cancers. Although doctors try to differentiate between a cancer and a benign liver tumor by performing blood tests and taking x-rays, sometimes the best approach involves repeating the tests in a few months to see if any change has occurred. Doctors usually avoid liver biopsies in a patient who is a candidate for a liver transplant because there is a small risk that the biopsy may spread the cancer.

Hepatitis C is the most common risk factor for hepatoma in the United States. Hepatitis B is a more common risk factor in other parts of the world where this infection is endemic. Other risk factors include cirrhosis from any cause, metabolic diseases such as hemochromatosis and Wilson's disease, and exposure to certain chemicals and toxins. Patients with hepatitis

C usually develop cancer only after the development of cirrhosis.

Patients with hepatitis C and cirrhosis should be screened for cancer on a regular basis. The goal is to diagnose a cancer before it has spread: The chance of a cure is higher in a patient diagnosed at an early stage. Once a primary liver cancer has spread outside the liver or is causing symptoms, the chance of a cure is much lower.

The American Cancer Society estimates that 18,510 new cases of primary liver cancer and bile duct cancer will be diagnosed in the United States in 2006. Most of these cancers will be hepatomas. The incidence of hepatomas has increased significantly over the last 5 years as a direct result of the increasing number of patients with hepatitis C progressing to cirrhosis. Hepatomas are even more common in the rest of the world, where approximately 1 million new cases are diagnosed each year.

The initial evaluation for liver cancer involves tests to determine whether a potentially curative surgical procedure such as resection of the cancer or liver transplant is possible. Patients who are not surgical candidates should see an oncologist to discuss other treatment options.

87. What are the signs and symptoms of liver cancer?

Liver cancer usually does not produce any signs and symptoms until the cancer has progressed to later stages. The liver is a large organ with few pain fibers and a large functional reserve. Liver cancers can grow to large sizes, invade blood vessels, and spread outside the liver before symptoms develop. In a patient with hepatitis C and cirrhosis, signs and symptoms of a cancer can be related to either the cancer or worsening cirrhosis and liver failure.

The following problems are potential signs and symptoms of liver cancer:

- Persistent pain over the liver or the middle of the stomach
- Unintentional weight loss
- Loss of appetite
- Feeling full after eating even a small amount
- Jaundice or yellowing of the skin and eyes
- Swelling of the abdomen or legs
- Internal bleeding from varices
- Worsening confusion
- A new blood clot in the portal vein

The development of any of these problems in a patient with hepatitis C and cirrhosis should prompt a thorough investigation for a hepatoma. Of course, the real goal in a patient with hepatitis C and cirrhosis is to find a hepatoma before the patient develops any of these signs and symptoms. An asymptomatic hepatoma picked up on screening studies is more likely to be curable.

88. Who should be screened for liver cancer and how?

Any person who is at risk for liver cancer should be screened on a regular basis. The exact protocol for screening is controversial, but most doctors use a combination of an ultrasound and a blood test called an alpha-fetoprotein (AFP) level. Patients with hepatitis C should be monitored on a regular basis for signs and symptoms of cirrhosis. Patients with hepatitis C and cirrhosis should be screened for liver cancer on a regular basis in an attempt to detect treatable cancer.

An ultrasound is an imaging study that uses sound waves to examine the liver and other internal organs. This noninvasive test is completely safe and does not carry any risks for the patient. In addition to screening for liver cancer, an ultrasound can provide other useful information, as discussed in Part 4, "Testing and Evaluation."

AFP is found in high levels in patients with a hepatoma. The levels of this protein do not rise in all patients with liver cancer, however. AFP levels also increase during pregnancy and in other types of cancers and can be abnormally high in patients with hepatitis C without liver cancer. In summary, an elevated AFP level can be seen in patients with active hepatitis C, and a normal AFP level can be seen in patients with a hepatoma. For these reasons, the results of an AFP test must be interpreted carefully.

No definitive protocol has been established for screening for liver cancer. Most doctors perform an ultrasound twice a year and perform blood tests (including an AFP level) every 3 to 6 months. Any significant finding is confirmed with a computed tomography (CT) scan or magnetic resonance imaging (MRI) scan. Patients with cirrhosis who experience any significant change in their condition should also be evaluated carefully.

Patients with hepatitis C and cirrhosis should be screened for liver cancer on a regular basis in an attempt to detect treatable cancer.

89. What are computed tomography (CT) and magnetic resonance imaging (MRI) scans, and when should one be ordered?

CT scans and MRI scans are radiologic tests that can take highly detailed pictures of the liver and other internal organs. These tests are ordered when initial screening tests detect an abnormality or if there is a high degree of clinical concern based on other factors.

A CT scan takes multiple x-rays of the body and uses a computer to generate cross-sectional images—that is, "slices" through the body. CT scans have been around for many years, and most hospitals have a lot of experience with them. A special contrast agent is injected into the patient's vein as the CT scan is being done. This agent helps differentiate blood vessels and can help distinguish hepatomas from benign liver tumors. In a small percentage of patients, the contrast agent may cause an allergic reaction. The contrast agent is also potentially dangerous to the kidneys, so it is generally not used in patients with kidney dysfunction. During the CT scan, patients are exposed to radiation, but the amount per x-ray is relatively low. Repeated CT scans may expose a patient to unnecessary radiation although the studies on this issue are somewhat controversial.

MRI scans use radio waves and strong magnets instead of x-rays to create pictures of the body. The radio waves are absorbed by the tissues of the body and released in specific patterns to create a detailed image of the body part that is being examined. A contrast agent is also used when examining the liver. MRI scans may be slightly better at finding liver cancers than CT scans. However, MRI scans are a newer technology, and some hospitals have less experience with them. MRI scans are more uncomfortable than CT scans and can be difficult for patients who are scared of enclosed spaces.

Whether a CT scan or an MRI scan is performed depends on the specific clinical situation, the doctor's preference, and the specific expertise of the radiologists who perform the procedures. Sometimes, both a CT scan and an MRI scan are done in the same patient when the information gathered by one technique is not absolutely clear. Although these tests are clearly superior to an ultrasound, sometimes they may not provide a definitive answer about whether a liver cancer is present. In these cases, the usual approach is to follow the patient closely and repeat the testing in a few months to see if there is any change. A hepatoma would be expected to grow over a few months, whereas a benign tumor would be expected to stay the same size.

90. What is the role of a liver biopsy if cancer is suspected?

A biopsy remains the gold standard for diagnosing any type of cancer. A liver biopsy allows doctors to obtain an actual piece of tissue from a liver mass and review it under the microscope. Although a biopsy is an invasive procedure, it carries a low risk of a serious complication. Liver biopsies are appropriate in some clinical situations but are not always necessary.

A liver biopsy may not be warranted when other strong evidence indicates that a liver cancer is present. This evidence should include a CT scan or MRI scan that is consistent with a hepatoma in a high-risk patient such as a person with hepatitis C and cirrhosis. An elevated AFP level greater than 400 milligrams per deciliter is also strongly suggestive of liver cancer when the CT or MRI scan shows a concerning mass. The risk associated with a liver biopsy in this situation is that cancer cells may spread via the liver biopsy tract.

Most transplant groups will not biopsy a high-risk patient with a clear mass who is eligible for a liver transplant. Instead, these patients are usually placed on the transplant list. A patient who is not a surgical candidate for transplant or resection is referred to an oncologist for other treatment options. Oncologists usually require a liver biopsy before they initiate chemotherapy or other treatments. There is less concern about spreading cancer cells in this situation because the patient is not being considered for a potentially curative procedure. If a biopsy in this situation shows a cancer type other than hepatoma, the treatment regimen will be adjusted appropriately.

91. What are the treatment options for liver cancer?

Proper treatment of a hepatoma is complicated and should involve a multidisciplinary team including a gastroenterologist or hepatologist, liver surgeon, oncologist, and interventional radiologist. Multiple treatment options are available, including surgical resection, liver transplant, tumor ablation, and chemotherapy. The correct decision depends on the stage of the tumor, the functional level of the liver, and the patient's general health. Some hepatomas develop in patients without cirrhosis. Most patients—including almost all patients with hepatitis C—have cirrhosis, however. This question discusses the management of a patient with hepatitis C and cirrhosis.

The first step is to assess the stage of the tumor and determine whether it has spread into blood vessels or out of the liver. The next step is to assess the level of functioning of the liver and any other significant medical problems. A person with early-stage cancer and compensated cirrhosis should be initially evaluated for a potentially curative procedure such as a surgical resection. Surgical resection is rarely considered in these patients, however, for two reasons. First, even with a successful resection, the patient is left with a diseased liver at risk for developing another cancer. Second, most patients with cirrhosis have limited liver reserve and there is a high risk of developing liver failure after the operation. These patients are therefore usually evaluated for liver transplantation.

Current national guidelines for liver transplants are based on a study from Italy and generally referred to as the Milan criteria. A patient is eligible for transplant if he or she has one tumor less than 5 centimeters in size or up to three tumors, all of which are less than 3 centimeters in size. There cannot be any invasion of blood vessels in the liver or any spread outside the liver. All candidates must have a CT scan of the chest to exclude any spread of the cancer to the lungs. Patients must also have a bone scan if there is any concern about spread to the bones. Part 11, "Liver Transplantation," discusses the liver transplant process in more detail.

If a patient is not a candidate for a surgical procedure, the next step is a referral to an oncologist. The oncologist will usually request a liver biopsy. Several treatment options are available at this point (Table 9), including ablative procedures (radiofrequency ablation, alcohol ablation, and cryosurgery) and chemotherapy (hepatic artery chemoembolization and systemic chemotherapy):

- Radiofrequency ablation involves the placement of a probe into the tumor and ablation of the tumor with radio waves.
- Alcohol ablation involves the placement of a probe into the tumor and injection of alcohol.
- Cryosurgery involves the placement of a very cold probe that destroys the tumor by freezing it.
- Hepatic artery embolization involves the placement of a catheter through the groin and into the artery that feeds the liver and the cancer. Particles coated with chemotherapy are then injected in an effort to reduce the blood supply to the cancer and to give directed chemotherapy.
- Systemic chemotherapy tends to be ineffective and poorly tolerated and is rarely used.

The oncologist will decide which approach is most appropriate in each specific patient.

Table 9 Treatment Options for Liver Cancer
Liver resection
Liver transplantation
Hepatic artery embolization
Radiofrequency ablation
Alcohol injection
Cryotherapy
Chemotherapy

PART ELEVEN

Liver

Transplantation

Can you give me an overview of liver transplantation for hepatitis C?

How are patients ordered on the transplant list, and what is the MELD score?

What are the risks of surgery, and what is the difference between deceased donor and living donor liver transplantation?

More...

92. Can you give me an overview of liver transplantation for hepatitis C?

Liver transplantation is a major surgical procedure that involves the removal of a diseased liver and its replacement with a healthy liver. The first successful liver transplant was performed in 1967. Transplant techniques have improved significantly over the last 39 years. In 2005, almost 6,000 adult liver transplants were performed in the United States. Most transplant centers report 1-year survival rates of at least 85 percent.

A patient with hepatitis C should be referred for a liver transplant when he or she develops liver failure or liver cancer. The basic thinking goes like this: A patient should pursue a transplant when survival is more likely with a transplant than without one. Most liver transplants are performed for patients with cirrhosis and a major complication. Other reasons for this surgery include congenital birth defects such as **biliary** atresia in children, hereditary diseases where the liver does not properly produce a protein, and benign liver tumors that grow to large sizes and affect the person's quality of life.

Transplant centers spend a long time evaluating patients; in fact, this process often takes several months. The evaluation process involves multiple tests of the diseased liver and the patient's general health. Patients also meet with many members of the transplant team, including a hepatologist, transplant surgeon, transplant nurse coordinator, social worker, infectious disease doctor, psychiatrist, financial coordinator, and nutritionist. The transplant team then meets as a group and reviews all of the information gathered during the evaluation. The team assesses the

Biliary

pertaining to the liver, bile ducts, or gallbladder.

severity of the patient's liver disease, the patient's general health with a focus on his or her ability to survive the surgery, and a psychosocial evaluation. The findings of the transplant committee are discussed at a follow-up appointment, and often more tests are required. The decision is often extraordinarily difficult because the current shortage of livers means that not all patients who need a liver transplant will get one. When a person is accepted for a transplant, he or she is placed on a list that is currently ordered by disease severity, with the sickest patients appearing at the top of the list. (A separate question discusses how the transplant list is ordered.) Patients are followed at the transplant center on a regular basis and contacted when a liver becomes available. Unfortunately, sometimes a person becomes too sick to survive a transplant and needs to be taken off of the list.

Hepatitis C is not a contraindication for liver transplant. In fact, it has become the most common reason for such surgeries, with some centers reporting that 50 percent of their transplant patients have hepatitis C. The concern is that hepatitis C returns in almost all patients after a transplant and can progress to cirrhosis in the new liver fairly quickly. Because hepatitis C decreases patient survival after transplant, doctors are actively looking for ways to overcome this problem. Treating and curing hepatitis C before surgery is the best solution, but obviously this effort is not always successful. Some patients are diagnosed late in the course of their illness and are too sick to tolerate the treatment. Hepatitis C can be treated after transplant, as described in a later question.

Hepatitis C is not a contraindication for liver transplant. In fact, it has become the most common reason for such surgeries, with some centers reporting that 50 percent of their transplant patients have hepatitis C.

The bottom line is that anyone with hepatitis C who develops liver failure or liver cancer should be evaluated for transplant. The transplant evaluation process may take several weeks to months, and patients often wait on the transplant list for a long time. Nevertheless, many patients are able to get a transplant and return to an excellent level of functioning and quality of life.

93. How are patients ordered on the transplant list, and what is the MELD score?

Many different systems have been used over the last 10 years to order patients on the liver transplant list. Every evaluation system is handicapped by the shortage of organ donors relative to the number of patients waiting for a transplant. In 2005, almost 6,000 adult liver transplants were performed, but there were more than 17,000 patients waiting for a transplant. Clearly, the order of patients on the transplant list influences who gets a transplant and survives and who does not.

The entire system is run by the United Network for Organ Sharing (UNOS), a nonprofit organization that operates the Organ Procurement and Transplantation Network under federal contract. UNOS has a very informative website that can be found at www.unos.org. Its listing system aims to place those patients who most urgently need a transplant at the top of the list. Organs are also distributed regionally, with the United States being divided into 11 regions.

The current system uses the **Model for End-Stage Liver Disease (MELD)** scoring system. MELD was

Model for End-Stage Liver Disease (MELD)

a scoring system that uses three laboratory tests (INR, creatinine, and bilirubin) to predict the risk of death from liver disease in a specific patient. This score is used to order patients on the liver transplant list.

originally developed to predict how patients would tolerate a procedure used to treat ascites and variceal bleeding. The score is calculated by a formula (available on the UNOS website) that uses three routine lab tests: the bilirubin level, the international normalized ratio (INR) level, and the creatinine level (see Part 4, "Testing and Evaluation," for descriptions of these tests). Subsequent clinical studies showed that this score is also helpful for predicting a patient's chance of dying from liver failure. Each transplant candidate is given a score ranging from 6 (less sick) to 40 (more sick) that predicts his or her chance of dying within the next 3 months. Patients are placed on the transplant list such that those individuals with the highest scores appear at the top. The list is also broken into blood types, although occasionally a donated liver may be given to a patient with another blood type.

The calculated MELD score is used for most, but not all, patients. The complete rules are complicated and beyond the scope of this book, but we will review some of the major exceptions here. Patients with a sudden and new onset of liver failure (called **fulminant hepatic failure**) have a very poor prognosis and are placed at the top of the list. This condition is rare and accounts for less than 1 percent of liver transplants per year. A patient with hepatitis C by definition cannot have fulminant hepatic failure because the liver disease is not new. Some patients in need of a transplant do not have liver failure so their calculated MELD score would be low and stay low, and they would never move to the top of the list. The most common example of this situation is liver cancer, where patients often have completely normal liver function and a low MELD score. The system assigns a higher MELD score to

Fulminant hepatic failure

the sudden and new onset of liver failure in a patient with no previous liver disease.

these patients and increases the MELD score every 3 months until a transplant is performed. A CT scan or MRI is repeated every 3 months to make sure the tumor remains within criteria for transplant.

The MELD system is not perfect in predicting which patients are most likely to die within the next 3 months but represents a major improvement over older systems, where variables such as waiting time influenced the waiting list order. Studies comparing the current system to older ones suggest that the MELD system provides an improvement in survival for patients waiting on liver transplant lists. Its other major benefit is that it is completely objective and allows direct comparisons between patients listed at different transplant centers. An educated patient on a transplant list always knows his or her current MELD score.

94. What are the risks of surgery, and what is the difference between deceased donor and living donor liver transplantation?

Liver transplant surgery is a major operation that carries both short-term and long-term risks. The long-term risks are mostly related to the medications required after transplant to prevent rejection; they are discussed in the next question. The surgery usually lasts 4 to 8 hours and takes place in three major stages:

1. The acquisition of the donor liver, which is often done at another hospital. The liver is then transported to the recipient's hospital in a special preservation solution.

2. The removal of the recipient's diseased liver, which involves an incision on the upper abdominal wall that is shaped like an upside-down "Y".

3. Placement of the donor liver into the recipient with reconnection of all the blood vessels and reconstruction of the bile duct system that drains the liver.

Patients usually remain in the Intensive Care Unit for several days and stay in the hospital for several weeks. Many complications are possible during the post-operative period, so patients are monitored closely. Immediate complications include standard post-operative issues including heart and lung problems. These are becoming less common as surgical techniques improve and patients are screened carefully. Complications that can develop during the initial hospitalization include rejection, in which the patient's immune system attacks the new liver; primary **graft** nonfunction, in which the liver does not function properly; infections; kidney dysfunction; problems with the bile duct reconstruction; and problems with the blood vessel reconnections.

Most transplants are done with a **cadaveric donor**— that is, an organ taken from a person who has just died. As mentioned earlier, there is a significant organ shortage, and techniques are being developed to help more patients on the transplant list get new livers. One increasingly popular technique is **living donor adult liver transplantation (LDALT)**, during which a portion of the liver from a healthy live donor is placed into the recipient. This approach is feasible because a healthy liver has the ability to grow back (regenerate)

Graft

a specific organ that is transplanted to another person.

Cadaveric donor

a recently deceased individual who donates his or her unaffected organs for transplantation.

Living donor adult liver transplantation (LDALT)

a liver transplant in which one person (usually a close family member) donates part of his or her liver to another person.

to normal or near-normal size. Both the remaining part of the liver in the donor and the donated part of the liver in the recipient regenerate to nearly normal size within several months. LDALT is not possible for every person waiting for a liver transplant. This complicated procedure carries significant potential risks for both the donor and the recipient. The decision to pursue LDALT requires thoughtful consideration and education of both parties and their respective families. Approximately 3,000 LDALT procedures had been done in the United States through the end of 2005. Studies suggest that survival in such cases is similar to that seen with cadaveric transplant if recipients and donors are picked carefully. The risk of death to the donor is estimated at between 1 in 200 and 1 in 5000.

95. How long are medications taken after a liver transplant?

Liver transplant recipients need to take medications for the rest of their lives. Taking the medications prescribed by the transplant team in the right amount and at the right time is essential to ensure the success of the transplant. The initial evaluation process stresses this point, and sometimes patients are rejected for transplant because of concerns that they will not comply with these requirements. Transplant recipients will be taking many different medications at the time of their discharge from the hospital after the transplant surgery. Over time, many medications are stopped but anti-rejection medications will be continued forever.

Anti-rejection medications help the immune system accept the new organ. Several types are available, and different combinations are used in different situations.

The types and doses used may affect the person's risk for developing recurrent hepatitis C, although the data on this point are confusing. Most of the long-term risks after transplant are related to these medications, so transplant doctors often try to keep the doses as low as possible after the new liver has been accepted by the immune system. However, these medications are never stopped, and taking them correctly is essential to the survival of the transplanted liver and the patient. Long-term risks include kidney dysfunction, high blood pressure, and certain types of cancers.

96. When should a patient be referred for a liver transplant evaluation?

In general, a patient should be referred for liver transplant evaluation when the likelihood of survival is greater with a transplant than without one. Hepatitis C patients are referred because of liver failure and liver cancer. Other individuals, such as patients with giant benign tumors, are referred for quality-of-life issues.

It is not always obvious that a person has a better chance of survival with a transplant, and the transplant committee will weigh many pieces of information when making its decision. Liver cancers need to be within certain criteria for transplant, so this decision is usually fairly straightforward. Patients with liver failure can have varying degrees of problems, and sometimes the team may decide that medical management or even a less risky surgery is a better option. In these cases, the transplant team will continue to follow the patient closely and may change its decision if the condition of the liver worsens. The MELD score is also used to help make the decision to pursue a transplant,

In general, a patient should be referred for liver transplant evaluation when the likelihood of survival is greater with a transplant than without one. Hepatitis C patients are referred because of liver failure and liver cancer.

although it should be used in conjunction with the patient's clinical condition. Some data suggest that a MELD score of 15 is a good cutoff, above which a transplant is a reasonable option. In many cases, however, the transplant committee would like to perform a transplant in a patient with a lower MELD score and believes that a patient with a higher MELD score is better off with his or her original liver.

The usual approach is to at least evaluate a patient once a significant clinical event related to liver disease has developed. For hepatitis C patients, here are the major events:

- Liver cancer
- Jaundice or yellowing of the skin and eyes
- Fluid buildup in the abdomen or legs
- Internal bleeding
- Episodes of confusion
- Worsening liver tests
- General failure to thrive with muscle thinning, malnutrition, and fatigue

97. Does hepatitis C come back after a liver transplant?

Hepatitis C comes back in almost all patients after a liver transplant. Because hepatitis C virus (HCV) exists outside of the liver in the bloodstream, essentially all patients experience reinfection of the new liver. The obvious exception is patients who have been successfully treated prior to transplant. The reinfection of the new liver is a major concern, and numerous strategies have been investigated to prevent or treat recurrent infection. The next question describes some of these approaches.

Recurrent hepatitis C in liver transplant recipients tends to have an accelerated course compared to the usual natural history of hepatitis C. Approximately 25 percent of patients will develop recurrent cirrhosis within 5 years of transplantation. This is significantly faster than the estimated 20 to 30 years that it takes to develop cirrhosis in a standard case. Studies have shown that 5- and 10-year survival rates are lower in HCV-infected patients compared to HCV-uninfected patients. Because retransplantation in these patients has a terrible success rate, many centers will not retransplant a patient with recurrent hepatitis C.

The reason for this accelerated course post-transplant is not clear despite extensive studies conducted by liver transplant teams. Multiple factors have been examined, including donor factors such as age, recipient factors such as race and sex, viral factors such as viral level, and transplant factors such as technique, presence of cytomegalovirus infection, and whether the patient developed rejection after transplant. One of the most intensely studied areas is the type of immunosuppression used after transplant. Hepatitis C recurrence appears to be more common and severe now than it was 10 years ago, which some doctors suspect may be due to the use of more potent immunosuppressants.

Patients are monitored closely after transplant for recurrent hepatitis C. Liver function tests, viral levels, and liver biopsies are followed to document return of the disease. The next question discusses what can be done when hepatitis C recurs.

98. Can hepatitis C be treated after a liver transplant?

Several approaches to the treatment of recurrent hepatitis C have been tried, but no standard protocol has emerged. The options include prophylactic treatment, pre-emptive treatment, and recurrent disease treatment. All of these approaches have risks and benefits.

Prophylactic treatment involves initiation of treatment at the time of transplantation with the goal of preventing recurrent infection. It is modeled after the successful use of hepatitis B antibodies to prevent recurrent hepatitis B infection. Several small studies have looked at giving hepatitis C antibodies to patients during the operation and the immediate post-operative period. Unfortunately, these studies did not show any benefit in preventing recurrent infection as defined by ribonucleic acid (RNA) tests. One study did suggest lower liver function tests and less liver biopsy damage, but these findings require confirmation.

Pre-emptive treatment involves early post-transplant treatment before there is evidence of recurrent disease based on liver function tests and a liver biopsy. Standard RNA tests will show evidence of virus in the blood. Pre-emptive treatment is typically started within the first 8 weeks after transplant. Many patients are not candidates for this approach because they are still recovering from the surgery and are too weak to tolerate treatment. Treatment regimens include interferon alone or combination therapy with interferon and ribavirin. Several studies have shown relatively poor cure rates for this approach, and it is not clear what advantage it offers over recurrent disease treatment. Pre-emptive treatment may be appropriate in patients who are at risk for severe recurrent disease although this outcome is hard to predict.

Recurrent disease treatment involves treating patients only if they have abnormal liver function tests and abnormal liver biopsy findings. Treatment of biopsy-documented recurrent disease is the approach used by most transplant centers. Patients are monitored with regular blood tests including liver function tests. Patients who develop abnormal liver function tests are referred for a liver biopsy, and patients with evidence of worsening fibrosis on biopsy are offered treatment. Treatment regimens include interferon alone or combination therapy with interferon and ribavirin. In general, treatment is poorly tolerated in post-transplant patients compared to nontransplant patients, with high rates of dose modification and treatment discontinuation being noted in the former group. Cure rates are also lower than in standard groups of patients.

In summary, treatment of recurrent hepatitis C after liver transplant is difficult, with no standard approach being used. Most transplant teams wait for recurrent disease as defined by liver function tests and a liver biopsy. Patients who are strong enough are then usually treated with interferon and ribavirin. Many patients fail treatment, but some patients are cured of infection. It is hoped that new treatment options will become available within the next few years.

PART TWELVE

The Future

Are there any new treatment options for hepatitis C?

What should I expect in the future?

More...

99. Are there any new treatment options for hepatitis C?

Current treatment of hepatitis C cures only about 50 percent of patients who complete therapy. Currently, intense research is underway to find new treatments. Researchers are studying the molecular structure of the virus, its ability to copy itself (replicate), and its differences from human cells. Finding drugs that effectively attack the hepatitis C virus (HCV) poses a difficult challenge. Hepatitis C copies itself with machinery that makes many mistakes or mutations. As a consequence, the virus is constantly changing, which gives it the ability to become resistant to our natural immune system and current drugs.

Hepatitis C treatment options can be classified into three distinct phases (generations). The first generation includes the currently approved medications interferon and ribavirin. These drugs were available before hepatitis C was discovered and were not specifically designed to fight HCV. While these medications offer a cure about half the time, many patients suffer side effects related to their nonspecific activity. These drugs cannot be offered to many groups of patients, including pregnant women or patients planning a pregnancy, patients with poorly controlled psychiatric problems, and patients with poor kidney function. Another drawback of interferon-based therapy is the length of treatment. Most patients in the United States require one full year of treatment. These medications are also expensive and require blood test monitoring.

The second generation includes medications that have been created to target specific areas of HCV and now are being studied in clinical trials. Most of these medications are aimed at the viral proteins NS3 and NS5B. The NS3 protein is essential for hepatitis C's survival because it enables the virus to copy itself. Drugs that inhibit NS3 are collectively termed protease inhibitors, because NS3 functions as a **protease**. The NS5B protein is also needed for replication of the virus—it copies the genetic code of hepatitis C from the virus's ribonucleic acid (RNA) code. Drugs that inhibit NS5B will target only viral cells because humans do not have this type of RNA code. These medications are collectively termed polymerase inhibitors. Several second-generation drugs are in advanced clinical studies and should become available within the next few years.

Protease

an enzyme that breaks peptide bonds between amino acids of proteins.

The third generation includes medications that have not yet been developed. Potential hepatitis C protein targets include p7, NS5A, and NS4B. For example, HCV copies itself on certain structures called membranous webs. Research has shown that NS4B may play a crucial role in creating these webs. NS5A may also play a role in replication with these membranes. Researchers are studying how these viral proteins can be targeted without affecting the human host.

Another potential advance in hepatitis C treatment will be the combination of drugs that target different parts of the virus. This approach should reduce the development of resistance and lessen the severity of side effects. Regimens consisting of multiple drugs have worked well in the treatment of other viruses such as human immunodeficiency virus, so we would expect that this will also be the case with hepatitis C.

100. What should I expect in the future?

Hepatitis C is a significant health issue for the United States and a problem that will probably increase in scope for at least the next few years. Its natural history requires 20 to 40 years to progress to cirrhosis and complications. Because many people acquired the infection in the 1960s and 1970s, there is a huge pool of people who have yet to develop clinical disease. A major goal of the healthcare system is to identify as many of these people as possible before liver disease develops and to treat them earlier rather than later. Doctors should ask about risk factors for hepatitis C and screen anyone with a risk factor.

The future is bright for hepatitis C patients, and we expect many new medications to become available in the next few years.

Hepatitis C patients should be referred to an appropriate specialist once the diagnosis has been made. Lifestyle modifications, including alcohol abstinence, are essential. Other risks for liver disease, such as obesity, should be addressed as well. Other medical issues that affect the ability to treat a patient, such as depression, should be treated. Every patient with hepatitis C should be assessed for possible treatment. Current treatments are not perfect, but they can cure many patients.

Researchers are actively exploring new drugs to treat hepatitis C. These medications target specific hepatitis C proteins and should be more effective in killing the virus with fewer side effects. The future is bright for hepatitis C patients, and we expect many new medications to become available in the next few years.

Resources

A variety of resources are available to patients with liver disease and their families. You can obtain a great deal of information from your primary care physician, your gastroenterologist, your hepatologist, or your local transplant center. Other resources are available through the Internet, though the quality of information on the websites varies widely. Here are some tips to help you evaluate a website:

- Check the "about us" section of the site. If no author is listed or no credentials are provided for the author, be suspicious.
- Check the attribution of the information. Experts have reviewed research in mainstream journals. Information from government agencies, such as the Food and Drug Administration and National Institutes of Health, has also been reviewed by experts. Information from drug companies may be reliable but remember, they are selling products.
- Information put out by patient groups can be biased toward one point of view.
- Be wary of emotional testimonials. They may be misleading or irrelevant to you.
- Read many websites and cross-check the information that they provide.
- If a treatment seems too good to be true, it probably is!
- Check with your primary care physician or gastroenterologist before making any changes in your treatment plan based on information taken from the Internet.

American Liver Foundation
(information, education, support)
75 Maiden Lane, Suite 603
New York, NY 10038-4810
Telephone: 800-223-0179
Website: www.liverfoundation.org

Centers for Medicare and Medicaid Services
Website: www.cms.hhs.gov

Children's Liver Association for Support Services
Website: www.classkids.org

Department of Public Health
(financial assistance)
Division of Organ Transplant Services
10 West Street
Boston, MA 02111
Telephone: 617-753-8130

Latino Organization for Liver Awareness (LOLA)
(information and education for Spanish-speaking individuals)
1560 Mayflower Avenue
Bronx, NY 10465
Telephone: 718-892-8697

Medicare
Website: www.medicare.gov

MedlinePlus
Website: www.medlineplus.com

National Council on Patient Information and Education (NCPIE)
(consumer's guide, information, education)
666 11th Street NW, Suite 810
Washington, DC 20001
Telephone: 202-347-6711
E-mail: ncple@erols.com

National Digestive Diseases Information Clearinghouse
Website: http://digestive.niddk.nih.gov/

National Foundation for Transplants
(fundraising information and short-term financial assistance)
1102 Brookfield Road, Suite 202
Memphis, TN 38119
Telephone: 800-489-3863
E-mail: natfoundtx@aol.com
Website: www.transplants.org

National Institutes of Health, Research Trials
Website: http://clinicaltrials.gov/search/intervention=%22liver+
   transplantation%22&recruiting=true

Glossary

Acute: Sudden or severe onset.

Albumin: A protein produced by the liver that accounts for most of the protein in blood.

Alkaline phosphatase: A blood test that measures injury to the liver or the bile ducts.

Alpha-fetoprotein (AFP): A blood test that is often elevated in patients who have liver cancer.

ALT: Alanine aminotransferase. See *aminotransferases*.

Aminotransferases: Blood tests that measure enzymes found in liver cells. These levels are often elevated in patients with liver disease. Aspartate aminotransferase (AST) and alanine aminotransferase (ALT) are the two most commonly measured.

Anemia: A low red blood cell count.

Antibody: A protein produced by the body's immune system to fight disease.

Antioxidants: Vitamins, minerals, and enzymes that reduce damage to cells by neutralizing free radicals.

Ascites: Abnormal fluid accumulation in the abdomen that can develop when the liver does not function properly.

AST: Aspartate aminotransferase. See *aminotransferases*.

Autoimmune hepatitis: A liver disease characterized by an overactive immune system that attacks the liver.

Bile: Greenish fluid produced by the liver that contains bilirubin, bile salts, cholesterol, and lipids. Bile flows through the bile ducts into the intestines, where it helps digest food.

Biliary: Pertaining to the liver, bile ducts, or gallbladder.

Bilirubin: A product of the breakdown of hemoglobin that is measured to screen for or to monitor liver or gallbladder dysfunction.

Biopsy: The removal of a small piece of tissue using a thin needle.

Bowel: Term used for both the large and small intestines.

Cadaveric donor: A recently deceased individual who donates his or her unaffected organs for transplantation.

Chronic: Usually refers to a disease that develops slowly and lasts for a long period of time.

Cirrhosis: A condition in which normal liver tissue is replaced by permanent scar tissue.

Coagulation: The ability of the blood to clot.

Complementary and alternative medicine (CAM): Alternatives to standard medical treatment that include supplements, relaxation, massage, and prayer.

Cryglobulinemia: The most common extrahepatic complication of hepatitis C, in which antibodies attack parts of the body and result in skin rashes, joint and muscle pains, and nerve and kidney damage.

Early virological response (EVR): Refers to the appropriate drop in hepatitis C viral levels that determines whether treatment should continue.

Edema: Excess fluid in the body that can cause swelling of the extremities and abdomen.

Encephalopathy: See *portal systemic encephalopathy (PSE)*.

Endoscope: Thin, flexible tube with an attached light that is used to view the digestive tract.

Endoscopic variceal ligation: A procedure using small rubber bands to treat varices in the esophagus and stomach.

Esophagogastroduodenoscopy (EGD): A procedure in which the esophagus, stomach, and duodenum are visualized with an endoscope.

Esophagus: The muscular tube that carries food from the mouth to the stomach.

Extrahepatic: A term used to refer to organs other than the liver.

Fulminant hepatic failure: The sudden and new onset of liver failure in a patient with no previous liver disease.

Gallbladder: A pouch connected to the biliary system that stores bile.

Gastroenterologist: A physician whose area of expertise includes gastrointestinal and liver disorders.

Genotype: A major strain of a virus. Because the hepatitis C virus is continually changing or mutating, six major strains of this virus exist.

Glomerulonephritis: Each kidney is made up of tiny structures called glomeruli that produce urine. In this type of kidney disease, the glomeruli are inflamed.

Graft: A specific organ that is transplanted to another person.

Hemochromatosis: An inherited disorder characterized by the abnormal accumulation of iron in the liver and other organs.

Hemolysis: The destruction of red blood cells.

Hepatic: A term used to refer to anything pertaining to the liver.

Hepatic hydrothorax: The accumulation of fluid in the lining of the lungs due to liver disease.

Hepatitis: Inflammation of the liver that causes cell damage.

Hepatocellular carcinoma: See *hepatoma.*

Hepatologist: A physician whose area of expertise includes liver diseases and liver transplantation.

Hepatoma: Cancer of the liver that often occurs in the setting of cirrhosis. Also known as hepatocellular carcinoma.

Hepatopulmonary syndrome: Low oxygen levels in the body due to shunting of blood in the lungs that occurs in the setting of cirrhosis.

Hepatorenal syndrome: A type of kidney failure that occurs in the setting of advanced liver disease.

Icteric: See *jaundice.*

Immunosuppression: Suppression of the body's immune system to prevent organ damage.

Interferon: A family of proteins that are naturally produced by the body and that fight off infection. There are three types: alfa, beta, and gamma. Alfa-interferon is used to treat hepatitis C.

International normalized ratio (INR): Also known as prothrombin time (PT). It reflects the body's ability to clot and is a marker of liver function.

Jaundice: Yellowing of the skin and eyes that can occur due to liver disease.

Liver biopsy: A test in which a small needle is passed into the liver and a piece of the liver is removed and then examined under a microscope.

Liver panel: A standard group of laboratory tests used to evaluate the functioning of the liver. These tests usually measure the levels of aspartate aminotransferase (AST), alanine aminotransferase (ALT), alkaline phosphatase, albumin, and bilirubin.

Liver transplant: A major surgical procedure that involves the removal of a diseased liver and its replacement with a healthy liver.

Living donor adult liver transplantation (LDALT): A liver transplant in which one person (usually a close family member) donates part of his or her liver to another person.

Living-related liver transplant: See *living donor adult liver transplantation (LDALT).*

Maintenance therapy: Indefinite use of peginterferon at a lower dose to treat chronic hepatitis C.

Model for End-Stage Liver Disease (MELD): A scoring system that uses three laboratory tests (INR, creatinine, and bilirubin) to predict the risk of death from liver disease in a specific patient. This score is used to order patients on the liver transplant list.

Neutropenia: A low neutrophil (white blood cell) count.

Non-alcoholic fatty liver disease: Liver disease secondary to excessive fatty deposition, often as a result of obesity.

Nonresponder: A patient who does not experience a significant drop in viral levels at any point during his or her treatment for hepatitis C.

Nonsteroidal anti-inflammatory drug: A drug such as aspirin or ibuprofen that has both analgesic and anti-inflammatory properties.

Palmar erythema: Redness of the palms; it occurs in cirrhosis.

Paracentesis: A procedure in which fluid in the abdomen is drained with a needle.

Partial responder: A patient who has a significant (100-fold) drop in viral levels, but never achieves an undetectable viral level, during treatment for hepatitis C.

Pegasys: A type of peginterferon produced by the pegylation of interferon alfa-2a.

Peginterferon: A type of interferon in which an inactive molecule called polyethylene glycol is added to standard interferon. This change increases

the length of time that the drug remains active against hepatitis C and allows for less frequent injections.

Peg-Intron: A type of peginterferon produced by the pegylation of interferon alfa-2b.

Pegylation: The attachment of polyethylene glycol to a protein.

Peritonitis: Inflammation of the lining that surrounds organs in the abdominal cavity.

Porphyria cutanea tarda: A blistering skin disease that affects sun-exposed areas of the body due to an enzyme deficiency in the liver. It may be precipitated by hepatitis C infection, iron overload, and alcohol use.

Portal hypertension: An abnormal increase in pressure within the portal system that usually develops in the setting of cirrhosis.

Portal system: Includes all veins that drain the small and large intestines, stomach, and spleen and that converge into the portal vein to drain into the liver.

Portal systemic encephalopathy (PSE): Confusion and mental status changes that occur in patients with advanced liver disease, most likely due to an increase in abnormal toxins.

Portopulmonary hypertension: High pressures in the blood vessels that enter the lungs in the setting of cirrhosis.

Protease: An enzyme that breaks peptide bonds between amino acids of proteins.

Relapser: A patient who has an undetectable viral level on blood tests performed at the end of treatment for hepatitis C, but a detectable viral level when blood tests are performed 6 months later.

Ribavirin: A synthetic antiviral nucleoside used in the treatment of hepatitis C.

Ribonucleic acid (RNA): A material inside cells that contains the genetic code for each specific individual. In humans, RNA copies carry the information from DNA out of the cell's nucleus. In the hepatitis C virus, RNA is the primary code needed for its replication.

Spider telangiectasias: Fine blood vessels on the chest and back that occur in patients with cirrhosis.

Spontaneous bacterial peritonitis (SBP): Infection of ascites; it can be treated with antibiotics.

Sustained responder: A patient who has a sustained virological response (SVR).

Sustained virological response (SVR): The standard definition of cure in clinical studies—hepatitis C is not detected in blood 6 months after the end of treatment.

Thrombocytopenia: A low platelet count.

Transjugular: Using the internal jugular (IJ) vein within the neck to access different internal structures. The IJ is used during a transjugular intrahepatic portosystemic shunt (TIPS) procedure and occasionally during a liver biopsy.

Transjugular intrahepatic portosystemic shunt (TIPS): Placement of a stent within the liver to allow increased blood flow through the liver. This procedure can be used to treat ascites or bleeding from varices.

Ultrasound: A diagnostic test that uses sound waves to evaluate internal organs.

Upper endoscopy: See *esophagogastroduodenoscopy (EGD)*.

Vaccine: A preparation of a specific weakened or killed virus or bacterium that is injected into the body to stimulate the immune system.

Varices: Dilated veins that are often found in the setting of advanced liver disease. They often occur in the esophagus and stomach and can rupture and bleed.

Wilson's disease: A liver disease characterized by abnormal retention of copper in the body.

Index

2013
Bruce~ A hard topic perhaps to
study, and worse yet to
have, but with knowledge
we, too, shall recover and
help all others !!!
— Your mom loves y